AF344484

MENSTRUAL CYCLE

SIGNS AND SYMPTOMS, PSYCHOLOGICAL/BEHAVIORAL CHANGES AND ABNORMALITIES

HUMAN REPRODUCTIVE SYSTEM - ANATOMY, ROLES AND DISORDERS

Additional books in this series can be found on Nova's website under the Series tab.

Additional e-books in this series can be found on Nova's website under the e-book tab.

OBSTETRICS AND GYNECOLOGY ADVANCES

Additional books in this series can be found on Nova's website under the Series tab.

Additional e-books in this series can be found on Nova's website under the e-book tab.

MENSTRUAL CYCLE

SIGNS AND SYMPTOMS, PSYCHOLOGICAL/BEHAVIORAL CHANGES AND ABNORMALITIES

MADELEINE GOSSELIN
EDITOR

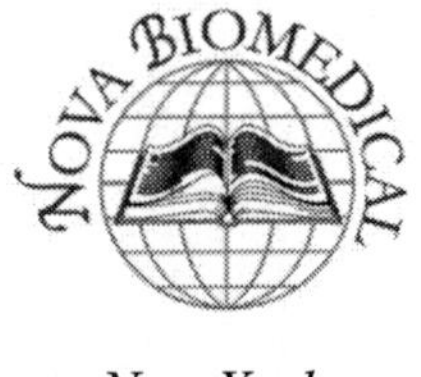

New York

NOTICE TO THE READER

Library of Congress Cataloging-in-Publication Data

ISBN: 978-1-62417-945-7
Library of Congress Control Number: 2012956451

Published by Nova Science Publishers, Inc. † New York

Contents

Preface

The menstrual cycle is the scientific term for the physiological changes that occur in fertile women and other female primates for the purposes of sexual reproduction. In this book, the authors discuss the signs and symptoms, psychological/behavioral changes and abnormalities of the menstrual cycle. Topics include the evolution of the menstrual cycle with a focus on the role of the luteal phase, extended sexual receptivity and the concept of concealed ovulation; functional and structural brain alterations associated with menstrual pain; premenstrual dysphoric disorder (PMDD) and premenstrual syndrome (PMS); the fluctuations on appetite and food intake that occur during the female reproductive cycle; and assessing energy intake and physical activity energy expenditure during the menstrual cycle.

Chapter I - The menstrual cycle has evolved relatively recently and is quite rare even among primates. Instead, most mammalian females have cycles of estrus. Distinguishing characteristics of the menstrual cycle have traditionally included: copious menses, concealed ovulation and extended sexual receptivity. The menstrual cycle consists of several days of menses, which is followed by the follicular phase, ovulation and then the luteal phase. The luteal phase, which is not present in many estrous cycles, is energetically more demanding than the follicular phase. Indeed, it has been suggested that a benefit of menses is that it helps the female conserve energy, by stopping the energetically costly build-up of an endometrium which cannot be fully re-absorbed. Bleeding is associated with reproductive cycles other than the menstrual cycle, but copious bleeding as a result of the sloughing off of the endometrium is unique to the menstrual cycle. In addition to the luteal phase and menses, humans and a few other species have extended sexual receptivity. Females with estrous cycles typically have a narrow window of sexual receptivity and in several species, the act of mating reduces that window.

This is unlike the extended sexual receptivity present during the entire menstrual cycle. Along with extended sexual receptivity, "concealed ovulation" has traditionally been thought to be a defining characteristic of a true menstrual cycle. However, converging lines of evidence suggest that although ovulation in primates may not be advertised, it may not be entirely "concealed," either. Not only physiological but behavioral and cognitive changes take place in the female during ovulation. Furthermore, behavioral and physiological changes take place in same sex as well as opposite sex conspecifics depending on the female's reproductive phase. This review will examine the evolution of the menstrual cycle, with a focus on the role of the luteal phase, extended sexual receptivity and the concept of "concealed ovulation" in women.

Chapter II - Dysmenorrhea is a widely presented gynecological disorder for women in the childbearing age. Females with dysmenorrhea suffer from disabling, cramping pain emanating from the lower abdomen with the onset of menstrual flow and the pain persists for 24–72 hours. Recent studies further disclosed that central sensitization exists in dysmenorrhea as hyperalgesia spans different spinal segments and multiple tissue systems (e.g., skin and muscle) and extends to non-referred pain areas during the menstrual phase. Moreover, menstrual pain is associated with functional and structural alterations in highly specified regions involved in pain transmission and modulation, generation of the affective experience, and regulation of endocrine function. The adaptive and mal-adaptive changes in the brain may be engaged simultaneously and dynamically and that some of these regions may underpin the hyperalgesia in dysmenorrhea. The functional and structural brain alterations may either be either state-related or trait-related. Where state-related changes are associated with the presence of menstrual pain, trait-related changes exist even in the absence of symptoms. When comparing pain and pain-free states, the rapid state-related structural changes in several regions correlating with the severity of the menstrual pain experience, suggesting that these changes are primary changes rather than epiphenomena. Some of the observed state-related structural alterations even persisted into the pain-free state indicating an accumulating effect of the cyclic menstrual pain. This notion is supported by a correlation of gray matter volume in these regions with menstrual pain duration. More specifically, regions involved in pain modulation and affect regulation exhibited hypertrophy and regions associated with pain transmission showed atrophic changes. Using positron emission topography to study state-related changes in glucose metabolism, the alterations in central processing of menstrual pain suggest that a disinhibitiondisinhibition of a thalamo-orbitofrontal-prefrontal network may promote central sensitization during menstruation. On the other hand, reduced metabolism was also found in sensory-discriminative areas, indicating a down regulation in pain transmission pathways. These findings are congruent with the structural brain alterations observed in dysmenorrhea. Overall, these results indicate that the adolescent brain is vulnerable to menstrual pain. Considering the high prevalence rate of dysmenorrhea and the early onset of primary dysmenorrhea, these findings mandate a great demand to revisit dysmenorrhea regarding its impact on the brain and other clinical pain conditions. Like the migraine, dysmenorrhea might be considered a chronic disease with episodic features but largely confined to the menstrual phase.

Chapter III - Premenstrual disorders include premenstrual dysphoric disorder (PMDD) and premenstrual syndrome (PMS). Unlike commonly occurring premenstrual symptoms, premenstrual disorders involve severe affective, behavioral, and physiological symptoms that cause distress and impairment. Research on purely biological causes for premenstrual diosrders has been unequivocal to date. Consequently, a promising area of research is to explore the role of psychological factors that may interact with physiological changes and contribute to the development and maintenance of PMS and PMDD. The current chapter focuses on psychological contributions to premenstrual distress, which are supported by the following: 1) symptom overlap and comorbidity between premenstrual disorders and psychological disorders, 2) premenstrual exacerbation of underlying psychological conditions, 3) the potential role of self-focused attention and coping in premenstrual disorders, and 4) symptom improvement as a result of psychological interventions. A holistic approach to premenstrual symptoms and disorders, involving biological, psychological, and social factors, provides a more comprehensive understanding of these disorders that has important implications for research and treatment.

Chapter IV - This chapter aims to review the mechanisms underlying the fluctuations on appetite and food intake that occur during the female reproductive cycle. These changes are the consequence of sex hormones variations during the menstrual cycle,cycle; therefore the effect of externally administered hormones will be extensively addressed. Estradiol has been deemed as the main hormone responsible for the reduction of intake during the periovulatory period. Activation of nuclear oestrogen receptors in brain areas such as the hypothalamus, hindbrain and reward system seem to be behind these effects. In addition estradiol also seems to increase the satiating potency of peripheral anorexigenic signals which leads to an early termination of meals. During the pre menstrual phase of the cycle intake is increased and although the underlying mechanisms are still not totally clarified, they point toward progesterone mediated antagonism of estradiol's effects. Externally administered sex hormones are the most common method used for birth control,control; they are also employed as hormone replacement therapy after the menopause and for medical purposes such as the treatment of menstrual disorders and endometriosis. In general these hormones are well tolerated; however, concerns about weight gain are amongst the main reasons given for the rejection or suspension of the treatment. Although this effect is commonly reported the evidence supporting this assertion is controversial. This review aims to provide a summary of the findings up to date on the effects of contraceptives on appetite and intake.

Chapter V - *Background*: Energy intake (EI) and physical activity energy expenditure (PAEE) have been previously evaluated across the menstrual cycle with food and physical activity journals. To the authors' knowledge, the direct assessments of EI, macronutrient intake, resting energy expenditure EE (REE) and PAEE have not been studied across the menstrual cycle within the same study design. Furthermore, no study has related these factors to possible variations in the severity of the premenstrual syndrome (PMS) and food reinforcement across the cycle. *Methods:* Seventeen women (Body mass index: 22.3 ± 1.6 kg/m^2; Body fat-DXA: $28.5\pm6.8\%$) participated in three identical sessions during distinct phases of the menstrual cycle: Early follicular, Late follicular/ovulation and Mid-luteal (confirmed by basal temperature and plasma gonadotropins, estradiol and progesterone levels). EI was measured inside the laboratory and under free-living conditions with food menus and food journals, respectively. REE and PAEE were measured with indirect calorimetry and accelerometers, respectively. Also measured were body fat mass (DXA), the severity of PMS, leptin and the relative- reinforcing value (RRV) of preferred foods. *Results*: No differences in body fat mass, REE, PAEE and leptin were noted across the menstrual cycle. Furthermore, no changes in measured and reported energy, carbohydrate, lipid and protein intakes, as well as the RRV of preferred foods were noted across the cycle. Differences in the severity of PMS (25 ± 10, 19 ± 11, 25 ± 10 points; $p<0.05$) across phases were noted. However, the severity of PMS and food reinforcement did not coincide with energy and macronutrient intakes. *Conclusions:* Taken together, these results suggest that the menstrual cycle may not be of practical concern when assessing food intake and physical activity patterns under the methodological conditions presented in this study.

In: Menstrual Cycle
Editor: Madeleine Gosselin

ISBN: 978-1-62417-945-7
© 2013 Nova Science Publishers, Inc.

Chapter I

Evolution of the Menstrual Cycle

Sharon Ramos Goyette[1,*] and Lincoln G. Craton[2]

[1]Department of Biology, Neuroscience Program,
Stonehill College, Easton, Massachusetts, US
[2]Department of Psychology, Stonehill College
Easton, Massachusetts, US

Abstract

The menstrual cycle has evolved relatively recently and is quite rare even among primates. Instead, most mammalian females have cycles of estrus. Distinguishing characteristics of the menstrual cycle have traditionally included: copious menses, concealed ovulation and extended sexual receptivity. The menstrual cycle consists of several days of menses, which is followed by the follicular phase, ovulation and then the luteal phase. The luteal phase, which is not present in many estrous cycles, is energetically more demanding than the follicular phase. Indeed, it has been suggested that a benefit of menses is that it helps the female conserve energy, by stopping the energetically costly build-up of an endometrium which cannot be fully re-absorbed. Bleeding is associated with reproductive cycles other than the menstrual cycle, but copious bleeding as a result of the sloughing off of the endometrium is unique to the menstrual cycle. In addition to the luteal phase and menses, humans

---

[*] Corresponding author: Sharon Ramos Goyette. E-mail: sramosgoyette@stonehill.edu.

and a few other species have extended sexual receptivity. Females with estrous cycles typically have a narrow window of sexual receptivity and in several species, the act of mating reduces that window. This is unlike the extended sexual receptivity present during the entire menstrual cycle. Along with extended sexual receptivity, "concealed ovulation" has traditionally been thought to be a defining characteristic of a true menstrual cycle. However, converging lines of evidence suggest that although ovulation in primates may not be advertised, it may not be entirely "concealed," either. Not only physiological but behavioral and cognitive changes take place in the female during ovulation. Furthermore, behavioral and physiological changes take place in same sex as well as opposite sex conspecifics depending on the female's reproductive phase. This review will examine the evolution of the menstrual cycle, with a focus on the role of the luteal phase, extended sexual receptivity and the concept of "concealed ovulation" in women.

Introduction

This chapter begins with an overview of the menstrual cycle in which we outline the hormonal fluctuations and mechanisms of action that control menses. In addition to menses, concealed ovulation and extended receptivity have both been considered hallmark characteristics of a true menstrual cycle. But the data we present overwhelmingly calls into question the notion that ovulation is concealed in humans. This essentially re-defines what has been a distinguishing characteristic of the menstrual cycle. We also examine extended receptivity and note that extended receptivity is not synonymous with continuous receptivity. Thus, continuous receptivity is considered within the context of the mating system that characterizes many human cultures. Theoretically, the adaptive nature of a menstrual cycle may stem from any of its features, some combination of them, or a combination of these features and other aspects of human social organization that evolved together as an adaptive "suite" (Lovejoy, 2009). Alternatively, the menstrual cycle or any of its components may be by-products of some other adaptation. It is from this perspective that we discuss the evolution of the menstrual cycle.

At this point, we present one notable caveat. The component processes of the menstrual cycle clearly have precursors in non-human primates. A detailed analysis of the phylogenetic distribution of the components of the menstrual cycle would thus be helpful in generating hypotheses about its evolution, but such a task is beyond the scope of this review. Consequently, in this chapter we focus on human data and draw only selectively from data on other species to evaluate what may be considered adaptive.

The Menstrual Cycle

The menstrual cycle differs from an estrous cycle in several aspects. Only a handful of species experience a menstrual cycle. Instead of a menstrual cycle, most mammals experience cycles of estrus. Cycles of estrus do not include the bleeding of menstruation, are typically confined to shorter durations and in many cases only occur during a breeding season. In most estrous cycles, ovulation is coupled to advertised sexual receptivity, ensuring that mating occurs when fertilization is most likely.

Estrous is derived from a word meaning gadfly and it described the behavior of cows that were driven crazy by these pests (Feder, 1981). This is similar to "hyster" which lends its meaning to both "hysterectomy" and "hysteria." These terms dramatize the changes in behavior that take place in most species during ovulation. In 1976, Beach identified three components of mating that change around the time of ovulation. These are attractivity, proceptivity and receptivity.

Attractivity is measured as the quantity of work in which a male will engage to gain access to a sexually receptive female. Proceptivity and receptivity, on the other hand, refer to the female's behavior. In many species, females do much to attract the attention of potential mates, around the time they are fertile. This includes ear wiggling in rats and sexual calls in primates. These are considered proceptive behaviors. Receptivity refers to the female's ability to actually mate. In females of most species, the physical ability to mate is coupled to ovulation. Receptivity that is extended beyond the window of ovulation is uncommon and receptivity that is continuous is rare.

Another major and often overlooked difference between the menstrual cycle and the estrous cycle is the level of variation within each (Burley, 1979). The estrous cycle remains quite fixed for a given species, for example, female rats cycle every five days; hamsters cycle every four days.

It is predictable. In women, on the other hand, the menstrual cycle length is not so predictable and the variability typically comes in during the follicular phase. (Oddly it is this component of the menstrual cycle that, at least functionally, in the ovarian cycle is most similar to animals with estrous cycles.)

Menstruation Does Not a Menstrual Cycle Make

The three defining characteristics of a menstrual cycle are: extended receptivity, concealed ovulation and copious menses (e.g. Butler, 1974; Burley 1979). For the majority of mammalian females, there is no menses, ovulation is advertised, and the ability to mate is tightly timed to ovulation. All of the physical, cognitive and behavioral processes associated with the modern human female menstrual cycle however, did not simultaneously evolve in our hominid ancestors. Instead, we find that only one aspect of the menstrual cycle, such as menses, exists in particular species. In another species, it may be possible to argue that the precursor of one or more components is present. For example, a few species here and there do show some aspects of the menstrual cycle, such as menses. Uterine bleeding has been documented in some bats (Rasweiler, 1992; Rasweiler, 2011; Zhang, 2007). However, bats do not have a menstrual cycle. Menses has also been document in the primates. The primates include the prosimians and the anthropoids. It is generally the case that prosimians do not menstruate. Of the remaining primates, the anthropoids, many have menses. Menstruation, alone, however, is not equivalent to a menstrual cycle. The extent to which concealed ovulation and continuous receptivity exist in species that menstruate cannot always be documented.

Many primates living in multi-male,multi-female social groups exhibit both visual cuesand specific receptivity calls during ovulation, making ovulation advertised, even if menses does occur (Domb and Pagel, 2001; Gesquiere, et al., 2007; Primate book). In chimpanzees (Watts, 2007) and baboons (Domb and Pagel, 2001 and Gesquiere et al., 2007) advertised ovulation is coupled with extended receptivity. So in some of our closest relatives, we have both menses and extended receptivity, but highly advertised ovulation. It is only in a few species, that we begin to see all of the components of the menstrual cycle emerging together.

Overview of the Ovarian Cycle

The ovarian cycle refers to the stages of development of the oocyte or egg. It involves the follicular phase, ovulation, and finally the luteal phase. The follicular phase is named for the follicle or group of cells that surrounds the egg or oocyte. The cells of the follicle work together to synthesize and secrete hormones, particularly estrogen, that are necessary for the maturation and subsequent ovulation of the egg. During the follicular stage, the follicle is stimulated to synthesize hormones in a manner tightly choreographed by the brain. The follicle itself becomes enlarged with antral fluid and will eventually rupture, releasing the egg. This is ovulation.

Even though the egg has been released, most of the cells that made up the follicle remain in the ovary. These remaining cells form the corpus luteum. Apparently, the corpus luteum received its name from its yellow-orange appearance under the microscope. The corpus luteum continues to secrete hormones. During the luteal phase, though, in addition to estrogens, progestins are also secreted.

The cells of the corpus luteum will undergo programmed cell death if they are not rescued by the hormones produced by a fertilized egg. The lifespan of the corpus luteum in the absence of a fertilized egg is typically 14 days. Therefore, in a non-fertile cycle, hormone levels decline because the cells that produce these hormones undergo programmed cell death leaving what is called a "corpus albicans" that no longer secretes hormones.

This also accounts for the finding that in women, the follicular phase is more variable than the luteal phase.

The Uterine Cycle and the Ovarian Cycle

The uterine cycle is dependent on the hormones (produced by the ovary and brain) that vary over the ovarian cycle. The superficial layer of the endometrium is particularly responsive to the sex steroids secreted by the ovary. During the first component of the phase, estrogens aid in the growth of the endometrium and then after ovulation, progestins, secreted by the corpus luteum cause the differentiation or "decidualization" of the endometrial stromal cells. The first phase of the uterine cycle during which the endomentrial cells undergo mitosis, stimulated by the high levels of estrogens secreted by the ovaries is termed the "proliferative phase." The proliferative phase coincides with the second half of the ovarian follicular phase. After ovulation, the cells of the endometrium differentiate and secrete a variety of molecules. Output from the endometrium seems to be highest about seven days after ovulation which coincides with the window of implantation. This component of the uterine cycle, called the "secretory phase," is under the control of progestins produced by the ovaries during the luteal phase.

The menstrual cycle refers both to (1) the complex interaction between the uterine cycle and the ovarian cycle and (2) the behavioral and other changes that occur as a result of the changing hormone levels. The menstrual cycle gets its name from the menses or copious bleeding that takes place if the endometrium can no longer be supported. This would only happen in the case of a cycle in which fertilization does not occur. On the other hand, if fertilization takes place, the fertilized egg remains in the fallopian tube. Seven to ten days after fertilization, the endometrium is "invaded" by the fertilized egg, which implants and begins the process of developing the placenta as a collaborative effort between the outermost layers of the blastocyst and the endometrium. This differentiation is considered "decidualization." The development of the endometrium in a way that maximizes implantation, should fertilization occur, is not unique to species with menstrual cycles. So the question becomes what differs between those species with endometrial decidualization but without menses compared to those that experience endometrial decidualization *with* menses.

The answer, in part, involves the progestin-induced differentiation of the endometrium. *It appears that in species with menses, decidualization is spontaneous, whereas in species that do not have menses, decidualization must be induced by the fertilized egg* (Dey et al., 2004). Decidualization appears to be induced primarily by progestins and elevated cAMP levels (Gallersen and Brosens, 2003). Among other things, decidualization initiates a whole series of changes in the endometrium that includes the recruitment of cells of the immune system (Yoshinaga, 2012). The progestins produced during the ovarian luteal phase enhance the cAMP/Protein Kinase A pathway (Gellersen and Brosens, 20003; Telgmann et al. 1997) and promotes the cytoplasmic retention of proapoptotic proteins such as FOXO1 (Christian et al., 2002; Labied et al., 2006.) Sequestering proapopotic proteins in the cytoplasm prevents their transport to the nucleus, where they would initiate programmed cell death. Essentially, progestins act as a barrier holding back the "bad guys."

But withdrawal of progestins, as happens in menstrual cycles in which fertilization does not occur, reverses the cytoplasmic accumulation and allows for the transport of FOXO1 to the nucleus where it initiates the synthesis of proapoptotic proteins, such as BIM, thereby promoting death of the endometrial stromal cells (Labied et al., 2006). To continue the analogy, when the progestins are no longer there to hold the bad guys back, death ensues.

Programmed cell death occurs in the endometrium, but that's not all. Most of our tissues are made up of cells connected together in a complex mixture of proteins and other molecules called the extracellular matrix. Progestins play a similar "holding back the bad guys" role here. High levels of progestins inhibit and progestin withdrawal promotes the expression of matrix metalloproteinases (MMPs) (Lockwood et al., 1998; Lockwood, 2011). MMPs proteolyze the proteins that make-up the extracellular matrix. Recall that the cells of the corpus luteum - that synthesize the progestins - undergo programmed cell death at this point in the cycle, if there is no fertilized egg. The net effect of this progestin withdrawal then is an up-regulation in the expression of enzymes that degrade the extra-cellular matrix. Thus, the endometrial stromal cells die and the extracellular matrix holding them in place is dismantled. The menses ensues.

Although the biology that explains many aspects of spontaneous decidualization (SD) has been elucidated, it remains unclear why spontaneous decidualization evolved. Furthermore, this is only one feature of a true menstrual cycle. In the next three major sections, we consider possible functions of menses, extended receptivity and concealed ovulation, respectively.

Possible Functions of Menses: Current Hypotheses

It has been suggested that the menses exists to rid the female's body of pathogens that exist in the ejaculate (Profet, 1993). However, several lines of evidence are in contrast to the predictions generated by this hypothesis. For example, pathogen load should be lower after menses and this does not appear to be the case (reviewed in Strassman 1996). It has also been suggested that the menses exists to save energy by initiating the end of the more energetically demanding luteal phase (Strassmann, 1996) but then we have to ask why a luteal phase exists at all.

The menses seems to have evolved in part due to an enlarged uterine size. Although several species experience a build-up of the endometrium, much of that can be reabsorbed. One key difference between prosimians which do not have menses and anthropoids which do have menses is the shape of the uterus. Prosimians have a bicornuate uterus, whereas anthropoids have a uni-chambered uterus (Martin, 2003).

This reflects the single births that are common among the anthropoids. Within the anthropoids several species have a menses that is "covert" or barely detectable. It is likely that these species represent a threshold uterine size, above which menses increases in correlation to endometrial build-up (Hardy and Whitten, 1987; Stassmann, 1996).

A By-Product of Spontaneous Decidualization?

Finn (1998) argues that menstruation evolved as a consequence of uterine changes produced by spontaneous decidualization. Clearly this is the case and the biology that describes this, as highlighted above, provides a proximate explanation. What is not clear is why some species with invasive placenta have menses and others do not.

In addition, if menses is a by-product of SD, then we need to address the question of why SD evolved. The *protection from fetal invasiveness hypothesis*, as described by Emera et al. (2011) views SD as one of the consequences stemming from maternal-fetal conflict, that is, the conflicting evolutionary agendas that arise because the mother and fetus do not carry identical genomes (Haig, 1993). This evolutionary arms race is evident, on the one hand, in the emergence of invasive placentation. This presumably evolved to benefit the fetus. On the maternal side, decidualization appears to have evolved to protect the mother against the invasive fetus. By this account, SD evolved because the fetus became increasingly aggressive in some species, resulting in so-called "hemochorial" placentation that allows the fetus to tap into the mother's bloodstream. In response the maternal decidualization reaction became more pronounced and preemptive--that is, SD evolved.

In contrast, the *embryo selection hypothesis* (Emera et al., 2011) posits that SD evolved to detect and act against impaired embryos at the time of implantation, thus limiting maternal investment in nonviable conceptions. This is plausible, given the high rate of chromosomal abnormalities in menstruating species with extended copulation, such as humans.

The *protection from fetal invasiveness hypothesis* and the *embryo selection hypothesis* are not mutually exclusive, and we believe they both merit empirical test.

A Useful Consequence of Menses

In an interesting study of a Hunter-Gather group, the Hadza of northern Tanzania, individuals were questioned about their understanding of the relationship between sex and pregnancy. Most individuals understood that sex causes pregnancy, but most also thought that conception is most likely to occur after menses. The author interpreted this as an indication that these individuals did not understand that conception is most likely mid-cycle (Marlowe, 2004). Other than right at mid-cycle, though, it is possible that "right after menses" could serve as a pretty good approximation of when fertility might be highest. Of course it is the case that one copulation on shy day after menses will not result in pregnancy. If, however, couples began copulating for several days, right after menses, it is likely that conception would occur. Many changes take place within the reproductive tract of women just prior to ovulation that collectively increase the window of sperm longevity. So, it is possible that menses could serve as a heuristic aid in the estimation of fertile periods. Also it remains to be determined if women universally understand that the menses indicates the lack of a pregnancy. It seems that having that knowledge - knowing that you are *not* pregnant- could be very useful.

Possible Functions of Extended Receptivity

Extended Receptivity, Continuous Receptivity, and Permanent Receptivity

Unlike most mammals that only copulate during a narrow window during ovulation or who ovulate only after copulation, humans and several other species copulate throughout the menstrual cycle, a trait commonly referred to as extended receptivity. In the literature, this human pattern is also sometimes called constant or continuous receptivity, and most recently, extended sexuality (Thornhill and Gangestad, 2008). It is important to distinguish extended receptivity and continuous receptivity. Several examples can be used to make this point. Firstly, there are species, such as the Lar gibbon and the Rhesus macaque, that have menses and in which sexual receptivity is extended beyond the window of fertilization, but not throughout the entire cycle (Hrdy and Whitten, 1987). This would be extended but not "continuous" receptivity. Secondly, in several species of baboons with menses and in which receptivity is extended or continuous throughout the cycle, copulations are not observed during pregnancy. In this case, receptivity is continuous throughout the cycle, but not throughout each reproductive stage of the animal's lifespan. These instances likely present evolutionary steps along the way to decoupling the tight hormonal control of synchronized ovulation and sexual receptivity. Therefore, it is useful to distinguish between extended receptivity, receptivity that is continuous throughout the cycle and permanent receptivity. We shy away from the use of the term "continuous" receptivity because that suggests an uninterrupted or non-fluctuating condition. Although not unequivocally established for every anthropoid primate species including humans, it does seem that there are fluctuations in copulatory activity. To make that distinction more obvious, we use the term "permanent" receptivity in referring to the human copulatory pattern to allow for the possibility of fluctuations in copulatory behavior.

Extended Receptivity to Prevent Infanticide

In most species, sexual receptivity (the ability to mate) is coupled to ovulation and therefore it makes sense to advertise ovulation. Importantly, in mammals, lactation will typically shut down the production of hormones necessary to promote another cycle of estrus. So while females are lactating they cannot mate again.

Many mammals exist in social groups that consist of several females. In this kind of social group, males compete for access to fertile females. A male who had been originally successful in competing for and securing exclusive access to the females in the group may be supplanted by another male at any time.

If females are lactating, when a new male takes over, the females will be physically unable to mate with the new male. Male behavior has evolved in response to this. Males will kill all the young of a certain age- or a certain time since the new male has taken over the group. This will shut down lactation in the females and allow for the resumption of the estrous cycle. In some species, the overtake by a new male, will actually induce spontaneous abortion in pregnant females. For the female, it does not make sense to engage in the costly and dangerous act of gestation and parturition, if the new male will kill the offspring. It has long been known that pheromones from a new male serve as the stimulus that induces spontaneous abortion in pregnant females in mice (Bruce, 1960).

Another way to counteract male aggression may be to extend sexual receptivity and advertise ovulation. For example, female chimpanzees who are ovulating, as assessed by sexual swellings, mate with as many males as possible (Watts, 2007) AND continue to mate throughout the cycle. It is thought that doing so confuses paternity and diminishes the likelihood of infanticide, consistent with the predictions of Hrdy (1981).

Flexible Mating Strategies

Before we begin the discussion on the possible advantages of human permanent receptivity, it may be helpful to make several distinctions. Firstly, as Dixon (2012) points out, it is helpful to think of primary mating systems and secondary mating systems. Doing this allows for a more precise discussion of actual mating dynamics. Inherent in this distinction, is the idea that mating strategies may be conditional (Alcock, 2009). That is, mating strategies may vary depending on the situation. For example, females in a polygynous social group may primarily mate with the single male in their group. However, if circumstances allow, that is, if a solitary male visits the group, which he may be more likely to do while she is ovulating, she may also mate with that new male. Her mating strategy varies with the situation. This is also consistent with another point made by Dixon (2012) and that is that the social system is not necessarily synonymous with the mating system. Thinking about mating strategies as flexible yields insights into the evolution of the human mating system.

Permanent Receptivity in Humans

Given that sex in internally fertilizing species is "expensive, dangerous, and time consuming" (Wallen and Zehr, 2004, p. 101), the modal pattern of a tight coupling between sexual behavior and fertility that occurs in non-menstruating species is easier to understand than the human pattern. Both females and males can increase their reproductive success and reduce risk by restricting sexual behavior to times when the female is fertile. This strongly suggests that, for humans, there is some selective advantage to non-reproductive mating.

In reviewing the evidence Thornhill and Gangestad (2008) come down strongly in favor of the *male-assistance hypothesis* which suggests that ancestral women's extended receptivity allowed them to gain nongenetic material assistance delivered by males.

Variations of this hypothesis have been in the literature on extended receptivity for some time (Buss, 1989; Hrdy, 1979, 1981; Symons, 1979) and seem to be the dominant view now. At first blush, this proposal would seem to be at odds with the notion that extended receptivity/concealed ovulation functions to protect female's offspring from infanticide by males by causing paternity confusion (Hrdy, 1981).

As Thornhill and Gangestad note, however:

> Though getting males not to kill one's offspring may not seem like obtaining "male assistance," by the logic of evolutionary economics it does, of course, qualify as nongenetic material benefit that increases female reproductive success and is "delivered" by males. In this sense, Hrdy's theory is a prime exemplar of the broader category of the "male-assistance" hypothesis. (p. 45)

Traditional explanations for concealed ovulation could also account for extended receptivity. That is, if concealed ovulation evolved in order to extend the male's investment throughout the menstrual cycle, it did so by encouraging males to remain with their primary partners and continue mating with them in order to assure paternity and avoid cuckolding. By this account, concealed ovulation and extended receptivity co-evolved as a strategy for promoting the pair-bond and male investment. There are several problems with this account.

Firstly, extending receptivity should INCREASE the female's opportunities for extra-pair matings, not decrease them! Secondly, this explanation confuses copulation with offspring. In many species of primates, males mate with several females. Each female does not receive benefits from the male, other than possibly protection, as in female defense polygyny. The female only derives significant benefits from the male when she has given birth to offspring. Furthermore, in some cases, the older female suppresses sexual receptivity in other females in polygynous groups. In humans particularly it is difficult to make the argument that copulation in and of itself engenders male assistance. The only case in which this does work is with infanticide prevention. In this case, copulation does indeed provide the benefit of preventing infanticide, as Hrdy described.

Then, it must be that male assistance is a benefit of extended receptivity only in species that pair-bond or are monogamous. However, there are species with extended receptivity that are not monogamous such as chimpanzees and the talapoin and Chacma baboon (Hrdy and Whitten, 1987). Furthermore, male assistance does not require extended receptivity. In several species, females are not continuously receptive and males invest heavily in their offspring (e.g. seahorses, California mice).

However, the most compelling evidence that extended receptivity is not necessary to engender paternal investment comes from studies of prosimians which have estrous cycles and are sexually receptive for only narrow windows around ovulation. In these primates, monogamy has evolved four times and the best predictor of paternal investment, a measure of male assistance, is whether the mother carries the offspring with her or leaves them in the nest (van Schaik and Kappeler, 1997; Alcock, 2009). In this case, the females do not have extended receptivity so this cannot support the male assistance hypothesis.

Given the immense maternal investment in offspring, there should be a strong evolutionary pressure that would favor conditions in the mating system that must work primarily on human female biology to foster the best possible outcome for the offspring. Maternal investment far outweighs paternal investment in humans. This is the case, beginning with the dimorphism in energy expenditure necessary to produce gametes and that difference becomes exacerbated during internal gestation. When body mass is taken into account, a comparison among primates indicates that women have the highest ratio of neonate mass to gestation period (Martin, 2003). When examining maternal investment beyond gestation women are still disproportionately higher than other primates. Mother-infant contact time between women of the !Kung is sustained at a higher rate than mother-infant contact in several non-human primate species (reviewed by Nicolson, 1987).

The *social affiliation hypothesis* (e.g., Wallen and Zehr, 2004) is a modification of a theory first proposed by Zuckerman in 1932. This makes the general claim that the selective advantage of non-reproductive mating in certain primate species is that it increases social affiliation between males and females. By this account, sex and attractivity "serve as powerful social cement," promoting "social cohesion," "social integration," and the "use of sex for multiple social functions" (Wallen and Zehr, 2004, p. 106).

Based on testes size and the middlepiece of spermatozoan, it is unlikely that sperm competition existed in our closest ancestors (Martin, 2003). Men, and male non-human primates have lost any "weaponry" (e.g. horns) long ago (Dixon, 2012). So, if males are cooperating and males and females are enjoying sex, then the social affiliation hypothesis seems plausible. Extended receptivity combined with not-so concealed ovulation creates a system in which, although mating may be taking place throughout the cycle, reproduction may be maximized by heightened female attractivity and proceptivity at ovulation.

This situation, which increases male-male affiliation and promotes male-female interaction, may heighten female-female aggression. The male might preferentially expend energy and highest quality sperm with his mate while she is most fertile. In this scenario, males may enjoy mating with their mate, but may also enjoy mating with other females.

Theoretically, this should heighten competition between women for the best mates, but since nearby females cycle together, all of the females are also most fertile and attractive and mating with their own mates during the synchronized ovulation. Altogether, this would simultaneously allow for mating during ovulation , while diminishing male-male and female-female aggression.

Concealed Ovulation... Revealed

Why Advertise/Hide Ovulation?

At least three explanations have been proposed to explain the benefits of advertising ovulation. Most of these explanations yield the greatest benefit if the mating system is polygynous. One hypothesis suggests that advertising ovulation increases male-male competition for access to the female, thus allowing the female to mate with the "best male" (Clutton-Brock and Harvey, 1976).

A second suggests that advertising ovulation ensures certainty of paternity (Hamilton, 1984) but this actually seems to support the most likely explanation, which is that each male who mates with the ovulating female could potentially be the father and this would diminish the likelihood of infanticide (Hrdy 1981). In chimpanzees, for instance, females who are ovulating (as assessed by sexual swellings) accomplish this by mating with as many males as possible (Watts, 2007).

Historically, the predominant view was that estrus was lost in human evolution and that ovulation became concealed. To explain concealed ovulation, a number of adaptationist theories have been proposed (for a detailed review of these and other accounts, see Thornhill and Gangestad, 2008). One influential hypothesis proposes that ovulation evolved to be "hidden" in order to extend paternal investment throughout the cycle, promoting the pair bond and paternal investment in offspring (e.g., Burt, 1992; Straussman, 1981; Turke, 1984). This account initially had considerable appeal.

After all, human pair-bonding and marriage are cultural universals, and characterize modern-day hunter gatherers as well. Contrary to popularized attempts to characterize humans as a promiscuous species (Ryan and Jethá, 2010), the evidence overwhelming suggests instead that we are pair bonders who engage in extensive paternal investment (Chapais, 2008; Saxon, 2012; Walker, Hill, Flinn, and Ellsworth, 2011). Other functional hypotheses propose that concealed ovulation secures food in exchange for sex (see Thornhill and Gangestad, 2008, especially Table 11.1, p. 271) but this has recently been shown to be improbable (Gilby, 2010).

One often overlooked hypothesis in regard to concealed ovulation is pregnancy avoidance (Burley, 1979). It is traditionally assumed that conspecifics do not "know" when a female is ovulating. Rarely discussed is that the woman herself does not "know" she is ovulating. Given our highly developed cortex, if ovulation were obvious to everyone in the group as well as the woman herself, she may avoid mating at ovulation to avoid the tremendous cost that accompanies pregnancy. The fact that so many humans at some point attempt to avoid pregnancy either through the rhythm method, hormonal contraceptives, barrier contraceptives or vasectomy and other such mechanisms does suggest that we are indeed a species interested in pregnancy avoidance, at least some of the time. This is true, even in our relatively privileged modern day society in which most healthy women do not worry much about the threat of predation, or death associated with pregnancy or birth, much less the scarcity of food. One imagines that our ancestors may have had even more reason to want to avoid pregnancy, at least some of the time, just as contemporary couples do. Given the tremendous female investment in egg production, gestation, lactation and beyond, it does seem quite plausible to think that pregnancy avoidance is a quite plausible explanation for concealed ovulation (Burley, 1979). Below we present evidence suggesting that ovulation is not so concealed, but the fact that the woman herself is typically not consciously aware that she is fertile, is undisputed and it may well be the case that this has the adaptive advantage of preventing pregnancy avoidance.

Only in a few species is ovulation advertised visually. The evolutionary history of humans is in part characterized by an increased reliance on visual cues and increased specialization of the brain for processing visual information. However, the absence of a visual cue of ovulation does not mean that ovulation is entirely concealed. Conscious awareness of a cue is not necessary for the cue to alter biology or behavior.

Instead, ovulation is typically "advertised" pheromonally and behaviorally. We will argue that both of these mechanisms of communication are still in place in humans. It is also noteworthy, that visual cues may still be in place in terms of sexual swellings. Certainly, estrogens and progestins affect the vasculature and it is possible that sexual swellings become more prominent in women during ovulation, but this may be visually obscured by pubic hair and/or bipedalism, and clothes.

At least as early as 1999, it was suggested that estrus may not have been "lost" and that ovulation may not be concealed after all (Pawlowski, 1999). Overwhelming evidence now suggests that ovulation in humans is not fully concealed in the traditional sense. On the other hand, it does not appear to be loudly advertised, either. Below, we survey the ways in which ovulation is, sometimes subtly, disclosed in human females as well as findings indicating that males are able to detect cues for ovulation.

Cycle-Dependent Changes in Women

Behavioral Changes

Behavioral changes in women occur around the time of ovulation in a myriad of ways. Compared to non-fertile days, women near ovulation are more likely to say yes when asked to dance by an attractive male (Guergen, 2009). Compared to low-fertility days, women try to look more attractive near ovulation (Durante, Li, and Haselton, 2008; Haselton, Mortezaie, Pillsworth, Bleske-Rechek, and Frederick, 2007) and plan to wear outfits that mixed-sex judges rate as sexier and more revealing (Durante, Li, and Haselton, 2008). Also near ovulation, women report increased interest in going out and meeting men (Haselton and Gangestad, 2006). Additionally, women's appetites decrease near ovulation and ranging activities such as locomotion and seeking social activities increase near ovulation (Fessler, 2003) which is consistent with estrogen regulated components of estrous behaviors in other species.

Cognitive and Perceptual Changes

Changes in the perception of auditory stimuli have been documented over the cycle. Women find deep voices in men more attractive when fertile (Puts, 2005) and this change in auditory processing even extends to changes in musical pitch perception over the menstrual cycle (Levitin, 2008). Interestingly, near ovulation, women show higher verbal creativity and fluency (Krug, Moelle, and Fehm, 1999; Symonds, Gallagher, Thompson, and Young, 2004), which may be influenced by changes in auditory processing, but may also facilitate behavioral interactions.

Although women's attraction to their primary partners does not appear to vary over the cycle, they report greater sexual attraction and fantasy about men other than their primary partners when they are fertile compared to when they are not fertile (Gangestad, Thornhill, and Garver, 2002). Because asymmetry in bilateral physical traits is an indicator of developmental stressors, symmetry is a reliable cue for good health in potential mates and the attraction effect holds especially for women whose primary mates are relatively asymmetrical (Gangestad, Thornhill, and Garver-Apgar, 2005) or lacking sexual attractiveness (Haselton and Gangestad, 2006; Pillsworth and Haselton, 2006; see also Bullivant et al., 2004).

Near ovulation, women rate the odor of T-shirts worn overnight by symmetrical men more positively than those of less symmetrical men; this is not the case when women are not fertile (Gangestad and Thornhill, 1998; Thornhill and Gangestad, 1999; Thornhill et al., 2003). When they are fertile, women report increased preference for men with masculine facial structure (relatively broad chins and narrow eyes) compared to when they are infertile (e.g, Gangestad, Thornhill, and Garver-Apgar, 2005; Johnston, Hagel, Franklin, Fink, and Grammer, 2001; Penton-Voak et al., 1999). Possibly as a by-product of their increased preference for faces with masculine features, fertile women identify faces as male more quickly when fertile than at other times (Macrae, Alnwick, Milne, and Scholoerscheidt, 2002) and show increased visual attention to attractive, as opposed to average-looking, men presented in a slide show (Anderson et al., 2010). Not surprisingly, though, near ovulation, women give lower attractiveness ratings to photographs of female faces (Fisher, 2004) which may be indicative of higher intra-sex competition.

This change in perception extends beyond the face. It appears that, in general, women have heightened attention toward male-related stimuli around the time of ovulation. Women find men who display confidence and act condescendingly toward other males sexier when they are fertile than when they are not fertile (Gangestad, Simpson, Cousins, Garver-Apgar, and Christenson, 2004). Women near ovulation pay more attention to products suggesting male conspicuous consumption presented in a brief (1 s) visual display than do women in nonfertile phases of their menstrual cycle (Lens, Driesmans, Pandelaere, and Janssens, 2012.) Near ovulation, women are more likely than at other times to report a preference for men with talent over men with wealth (Haselton and Miller, 2006) as short-term mates, and they find men judged to be faithful as less sexy (Thornhill et al., 2003).

Physical Changes

Physical changes take place in odor, face and body symmetry and voice during the cycle, and these can be detected by men. Based on male response, a women's scent appears to change when she is ovulating. Men rate women's odor more positively at high compared to low fertility periods, as measured with samples of vaginal secretions (Doty et al., 1975), or using T-shirts worn overnight by women (Thornhill et al., 2003; see also Havlíček, Dvořáková, Bartoš, and Flegr, 2006; Kuukasiarvi et al., 2004; Singh and Bronstad, 2001). Female voices are higher in pitch (Bryant and Haselton, 2009) and rated more positively by mixed-sex judges (Pipitone and Gallup, 2008) when recorded at high fertility than at low fertility.

The qualitative value of a woman's physical attractiveness is also assessed differently depending on where she is in the cycle. Women's faces may become subtly more attractive near ovulation (Roberts et al., 2004), and their bodies increase in soft-tissue body symmetry (Manning, Scutt, Whitehouse, Leinster, and Walton, 1996) and decrease in waist-to-hip ratio (Kirchengast and Gartner, 2002; see also Singh and Bronstad, 2001, Thornhill et al., 2003). It is not yet clear whether women are aware of their increased attractiveness at ovulation, but if so, it may help explain their increased interest in self-ornamentation—this would be a time to "advertise" both to potential mates but also to nearby conspecifics.

Cycle-Dependent Changes in Other Women

As McClinock's elegant studies (1971, 1998) have demonstrated, pheromones from women can shift the menstrual cycles of other nearby women. Her ground-breaking work originally demonstrated the synchrony of cycling in women who lived together in dorms (1971). Her later work revealed that pheromones mediate this effect (1998). Axillary (or underarm) secretions were swabbed from women during either the luteal or follicular phase of their menstrual cycles.

These were then placed on the upper lip of other women. It was found that if the recipient was exposed to secretions during the follicular phase, her pre-ovulatory lutenizing hormone (LH) surge was phase advanced. If instead the secretions were from the luteal phase, then the recipient's LH surge was delayed, lengthening her cycle. So, in the post-pubescent female, the menstrual cycle is malleable.

Other work shows that individuals living nearby can alter the onset of puberty. Additional studies show the effect of the presence of the biological father or older sisters on shifting the onset of puberty (Deardorff, 2011).

Cycle-Dependent Changes in Men

Each of the cycle-dependent behavioral, cognitive/ perceptual, and physical changes in women summarized above is potentially detectable by men. The emerging evidence indicates that men can detect ovulation.

Behavioral Changes

Mate guarding behavior changes over the cycle. Women's reports of their romantic partner's behavior taken across their menstrual cycle indicate that they perceive their partners to be more attentive, vigilant, or monopolizing when the women are near ovulation (Gangestad, et al., 2002). This effect is strongest for relationships that were not yet steady or exclusive. Women also perceive their partners to be more loving or spoiling (Gangestad, et al., 2002; Haselton and Gangestad, 2006; Pillsworth and Haselton, 2006) and more jealous and possessive (Haselton and Gangestad, 2006; Pillsworth and Haselton, 2006) when the women are near ovulation. The fact that this behavior is related to mating opportunities is underscored by the finding that less-attractive men increase their mate guarding during their partner's fertility more than attractive men do. More-attractive women are mate guarded all the time, but less-attractive women are especially guarded when fertile (Haselton and Gangestad, 2006).

Cognitive/Perceptual Changes

Each of the cycle-dependent behavioral, cognitive/ perceptual, and physical changes in women summarized above is potentially detectable by men. The emerging evidence indicates that men can detect ovulation. Changes in the behavior of the male in response to ovulation support this point. In an astounding experiment, Miller, Tybur and Jordan (2007) reported that regularly ovulating women working as lap dancers earned significantly more in tips near the time they were ovulating than at other times during the menstrual cycle.

Physical Changes

As mentioned above, men rate women's odor more positively at high than at low fertility, as measured with samples of vaginal secretions (Doty et al., 1975), or using T-shirts worn overnight by women (Thornhill et al., 2003, Singh and Bronstad, 2001). In one study showing the truly socio-endocrinological (Bercovitch and Ziegler, 1990) nature of the menstrual cycle, men responded to physiological changes in women with a physiological change of their own. Men exposed to body odor samples of women have higher testosterone in response to samples taken from high fertility women than for samples taken from low fertility women (Miller and Maner, 2010).

Implications of Cycle-Dependent Changes and Men's Detection of Them

The rapidly growing literature summarized above is revealing that estrus has not, in fact, been lost, that ovulation is not fully concealed, and that men appear to be sensitive to many of the available cues for ovulation. In their review, Haselton and Gildersleeve (2011) offer three evolutionary hypotheses to account for these data:

The *signaling hypothesis* proposes that cycle-dependent changes in women are advertisements, that is, cues designed to signal fertility.

The *leaky cues hypothesis* proposes that selection pressures have worked to conceal ovulation, but that concealment is necessarily imperfect and men have evolved counterstrategies that allow them to detect subtle cues.

The *female quality hypothesis* proposes cycle-dependent changes in women's attractiveness are an incidental by-product of an adaptation that is designed to signal mate quality differences between women. The notion is that women signal their mate quality via her estrogen levels and resulting changes such as in odor and vocal quality. Because estrogen levels vary within as well as between women, however, cycle-dependent changes in attractiveness occur.

Conclusion

Signalling, Leaky Cues, or By-Product?

The recent work reviewed in the previous section makes it clear that ovulation is not, strictly speaking, concealed. Consequently, we need a theory of the human menstrual cycle that accounts for not-so-well-concealed ovulation, the physiological and cognitive changes it causes in conspecifics, permanent receptivity and menses. The signalling, leaky cues, and female quality hypotheses three hypotheses stated above can serve as a starting point.

The signaling hypothesis has been questioned on several grounds (Thornhill and Gangestad, 2008). Basically, it would decrease female choice.

If women signal their fertility they are likely to attract the attention of all men, including those of low genetic quality. However, if correct, this hypothesis also raises the interesting question of why advertisement appears to be so subtle in humans as compared to other species for whom fertility is loudly advertised, for instance in salient sexual swellings.

If the leaky cues hypothesis is correct, then selection pressures have worked to conceal ovulation. It is just imperfectly concealed. This account must explain why estrus has been retained but cues for it are being hidden.

Researchers are bound to find it difficult to tease apart the signaling and leaky cues hypotheses. Both fertile women seeking "good genes" outside their primary partnerships and extra-pair males possessing those good genes would benefit reproductively if cues for ovulation are subtle enough to avoid straightforward detection by women's primary partners. As Miller et al. (2007) eloquently state, "We suspect that human estrous cues are likely to be very flexible and stealthy—subtle behavioral signals that fly below the radar of conscious intention or perception, adaptively hugging the cost-benefit contours of opportunistic infidelity" (p. 380).

Dual Sexual Strategy Theory: State of the Art?

In order to account for both the subtly of ovulation cues and the fact of extended receptivity (among other things), Thornhill and Gangestad (2008) recently propose a *dual sexual strategy account*:

> Women have two functionally distinct sexualities. Estrus functions to identify good sires (which may or may not be the primary partner). Extended sexuality functions to secure nongenetic material benefits from males. Women's extended-sexuality mate preferences possess design features different from estrous mate preferences. Although women's preferences for stable pair-bond partners are stable across the cycle (and function to favor both genetic and material benefits), women's preferences for sex partners during estrus focus on traits that connote possession of good genes. (p. 324)

The dual sexual strategy account makes three major claims: 1) Sexuality at peak fertility evolved to make it possible for women to mate with males possessing "good genes"; 2) "cues" for fertility that make females more attractive to males in the fertile phase of the menstrual cycle are not signals of fertility but rather by-products of changes in the female's reproductive physiology; and 3) extended receptivity evolved in order to obtain nongenetic material benefits from males.

The first claim is supported in particular by evidence, reviewed above, consistent with the so-called *ovulatory-shift hypothesis* (Gangestad, Thronhill, Garver-Apgar, 2005). This proposes that changes in female mate preferences and sexual interests shift adaptively during the menstrual cycle. In particular, it regards mating with short-term sex partners with "good genes" as being most reproductively beneficial during fertility. When infertile, this is potentially too costly because it may lead to loss of a long term social mate without the possibility of reaping any reproductive benefit. In addition to changes in mate preferences and sexual interests that might serve to advertise and adaptively exploit their fertility, women display other cycle-dependent behavioral, cognitive, and physical changes that make them particularly attractive to potential mates near ovulation.

The ovulatory-shift hypothesis predicts that near ovulation, women will be more attracted than at other times to "sexy" male traits in men other than their long term partners.

As we have seen, this is indeed the case. Near ovulation, women are more attracted to men with physical traits such as masculine faces, and behavioral traits such as competitive behavior, and to men who are not their primary partners. The latter is especially true for women whose primary partners lack these traits.

The second claim above seems more tentative to us. It predicts that all the morphological, vocal or other female traits that become more attractive to males in the fertile phase of the menstrual cycle are incidental by-products of changes in the female's physiology (and therefore are not signals selected by evolution). Thus, Thornhill and Gangestad clearly side with the leaky cues hypothesis stated above, arguing that "Women possess estrus, but they also possess adaptations to conceal it" (2008, p. 327).

Thornhill and Ganstead's (2008) account of women's sexual behavior when fertile, as summarized in the first two claims above, also points to some other new hypotheses. For instance, they speculate that decreased appetite near ovulation (Fessler, 2003) might do more than simply function to motivate ancestral women to mate rather than forage. It might in fact help women not be tempted to trade sex for food offered by men with "poor genes" but the "food for sex" hypothesis is not supported by data.

The dual sexual strategy account portrays human sexuality, and the menstrual cycle, as an evolutionary arms race between the genders. In evolutionary terms, it would be advantageous for men to be able to detect ovulation, since mating during the narrow window of ovulation would reap the most reproductive benefits. In addition, awareness of a partner's fertility makes it possible to deter her extra-pair mating when it would be most likely to lead to conception. Thus, as selection pressures push women to conceal ovulation, selection pressures on males push them to attune to whatever subtle cues are "leaked." Thornhill and Gangestad (2008) regard their view as provisional, and other logical possibilities certainly exist. For instance, the female quality hypothesis for concealed ovulation is quite plausible. Possibly, ovulation *per se* is neither advertised nor concealed! That is, these cues might not reflect evolved signals but rather "detectable by-products" of female physiological changes that lead to ovulation, particularly changes stemming from increases in estrogen. This view does see estrogen levels and associated traits as advertisement, but as advertisement for overall quality of the individual female, not advertisement for ovulation.

As we have already spent a good deal of time discussing, the data suggest that it is implausible that a potential gain of non-genetic benefits was the evolutionary factor that promoted extended receptivity. Data on the prosimians which do NOT have extended receptivity, but in which there is high paternal investment argue directly against this position. More recently a direct test of a non-genetic benefit, e.g. food-for-mating, was carried out in chimpanzees (Gilby et al., 2010). These data also argue against the male assistance hypothesis. Instead, the available data suggest that the answer is more complex and more inclusive. We must evaluate many aspects of our social structure, conditional mating strategies and our primary mating system of monogamy if we are to understand the benefits of the menstrual cycle. We must consider a suite of factors influencing the evolution of the menstrual cycle: our diminished physical sexual dimorphism, limited intra- and intersex aggression, a comparative lack of dependence of mating on hormones in men and women, the fact that the reproductive cycles of women impact the reproductive cycles of other women and the physiology of men, and our very altricial young. Together, these factors suggest a socioendocrinological perspective from which to examine the benefits of the menstrual cycle.

The Adaptable Menstrual Cycle: A Socioendocrinological Perspective

A socioendocrinological perspective emphasizes the importance of the social group on the reproductive success of individual members. In this view, permanent receptivity, unknowingly advertised ovulation that can modulate behavior and fertility in nearby same and opposite sex conspecifics, and a prolonged luteal phase with spontaneous decidualization and menses, have evolved in our bipedal, large-brained, single-birth, mostly monogamous social species to promote the survival of our very altricial offspring to an age at which reproductive success is possible. Thus the data suggest that the menstrual cycle is not fixed, but malleable and changes with varying social contexts.

This kind of shift in thinking can impact very real and contemporary problems. For example, thinking about the menstrual cycle from a socioendocrinological perspective directly opens up avenues for novel hypotheses regarding the increasingly younger age at which girls are entering menarche.

Obesity and BMI have been implicated and certainly BMI affects the onset of puberty in girls, but this is not the whole story. Comparisons of age of menarche between US and Denmark populations suggest that BMI is only part of the story (Juul, Teilman et al., 2006). The pubertal status of 1,100 girls in Denmark was compared to the pubertal status of girls in Denmark from 1964. While the researchers did find that BMI was negatively correlated with age of onset of puberty, they found no overall decrease in the average age of onset of puberty in girls, similar to studies from Italy (Russo et al., 2012, Rigon, 2012), but unlike studies from the US (Euling, et al., 2008, Herman-Giddens, 2006).

Research is now accumulating to suggest that an antecedent of early menarche is the absence the father (Bogaert, 2005; Matchock and Susman, 2006; Deardorff et al., 2011). Other socioendocrinological factors have also been implicated such as income (Deardoff et al., 2011) and neighborhood dynamics (Deardorff et al., 2012). When a young girl enters precocious menarche she is at increased risk for a myriad of health issues including: ovarian cancer (Gong et al., 2012), metabolic syndrome (Akter, et al., 2012), anxiety disorders (Weingarden, Renshaw, 2012) as well as others. Additionally, an earlier age of onset of puberty might lead to decisions or behaviors that are disadvantageous.

For example, the age at which girls/women begin taking the pill leads to an earlier age of a diagnosis of breast cancer (Imkampe and Bates, 2012). Recent guidelines have suggested lowering the age of precocious menarche to an absurdly young age (Kaplowitz and Oberfield, 1999) which has wisely been challenged (Midyett, Moore and Jacobson, 2003; Sorensen, 2012). When we consider the menstrual cycle from a socioendocrinological perspective, instead of mindlessly dismissing the epidemic of precocious puberty and all of the associated health issues to which it predisposes our girls as a biological *fete accompli* and adjusting the age of diagnosis, we might instead consider the factors that are causing this and then develop solutions around those data.

In conclusion, we suggest considering the menstrual cycle to be a complex, malleable phenomenon capable of responding to an ever-changing interdependent social and biological milieu. Such a re-framing is perhaps overdue.

Acknowledgments

The authors would like to thank Theresa Lynn for assistance in gathering sources and in constructing the reference section, Nicole Capezza for suggesting primary sources, and John McCoy for helpful comments on a draft of the manuscript.

References

Akter, S., Jesmin, S., Islam, M., Sultana, S. N., Okazaki, O., Hiroe, M., Mizutani, T. (2012). Association of age at menarche with metabolic syndrome and its components in rural bangladeshi women. *Nutrition and Metabolism, 9*(1), 99. doi: 10.1186/1743-7075-9-99.

Alcock, J. (2009). *Animal behavior* (9th ed.). Sunderland, Massachusetts: Sinauer Associates, Inc.

Anderson, U. S., Perea, E. F., Becker, D. V., Ackerman, J. M., Shapiro, J. R., Neuberg, S. L., and Kenrick, D. T. (2010). I only have eyes for you: Ovulation redirects attention (but not memory) to attractive men. *Journal of Experimental Social Psychology, 46*(5), 804-808. doi: 10.1016/j.jesp. 2010.04.015.

Beach, F. A. (1976). Sexual attractivity, proceptivity, and receptivity in female mammals. *Hormones and Behavior, 7*(1), 105-138.

Bercovitch, F. B. and Ziegler, T. E. (1990). Introduction to socioendocrinology. In: F. B. Bercovitch and T. E. Ziegler (Eds.), *Socioendocrinology of primate reproduction* (pp. 1-9). New York: Wiley-Liss.

Blaffer Hrdy, S. and Whitten, P. L. (1987). Patterning of sexual activity. In: B. B. Smuts, D. L. Cheney, R. M. Seyfarth, R. W. Wrangham and T. T.

Struhsaker (Eds.), *Primate societies* (pp. 370-384). Chicago and London: The University of Chicago Press.

Bogaert, A. F. (2005). Age at puberty and father absence in a national probability sample. *Journal of Adolescence, 28*(4), 541-546. doi: 10.1016/ j.adolescence.2004.10.008

Bruce, H. M. (1960). A block to pregnancy in the mouse caused by proximity of strange males. *Journal of Reproduction and Fertility, 1*, 96-103.

Bryant, G. A. and Haselton, M. G. (2009). Vocal cues of ovulation in human females. *Biology Letters, 5*(1), 12-15. doi: 10.1098/rsbl.2008.0507

Bullivant, S. B., Sellergren, S. A., Stern, K., Spencer, N. A., Jacob, S., Mennella, J. A., and McClintock, M. K. (2004). Women's sexual experience during the menstrual cycle: Identification of the sexual phase by noninvasive measurement of luteinizing hormone. *Journal of Sex Research, 41*(1), 82-93. doi: 10.1080/00224490409552216

Burt, A. (1992). 'Concealed ovulation' and sexual signals in primates. *Folia Primatologica; International Journal of Primatology, 58*(1), 1-6.

Chapais, B. (2008). *Primeval kinship: How pair-bonding gave birth to human society*. Cambridge, MA: Harvard University Press.

Clutton-Brock, T. H. and Harvey, P. H. (1976). Evolutionary rules and primate societies. In: P. P. G. Batson and R. A. Hinde (Eds.), *Growing points in ethology* (pp. 195-238). Cambrigde: Cambridge University Press.

Deardorff, J., Ekwaru, J. P., Kushi, L. H., Ellis, B. J., Greenspan, L. C., Mirabedi, A., Hiatt, R. A. (2011). Father absence, body mass index, and pubertal timing in girls: Differential effects by family income and ethnicity. *The Journal of Adolescent Health: Official Publication of the Society for Adolescent Medicine, 48*(5), 441-447. doi: 10.1016/j. jado health.2010.07.032.

Deardorff, J., Fyfe, M., Ekwaru, J. P., Kushi, L. H., Greenspan, L. C., and Yen, I. H. (2012). Does neighborhood environment influence girls' pubertal onset? Findings from a cohort study. *BMC Pediatrics, 12*, 27-2431-12-27. doi: 10.1186/1471-2431-12-27; 10.1186/1471-2431-12-27

Domb, L. G. and Pagel, M. (2001). Sexual swellings advertise female quality in wild baboons. *Nature, 410*(6825), 204-206. doi: 10.1038/35065597.

Doty, R. L., Ford, M., Preti, G., and Huggins, G. R. (1975). Changes in the intensity and pleasantness of human vaginal odors during the menstrual cycle. *Science (New York, N.Y.), 190*(4221), 1316-1318.

Durante, K. M., Li, N. P. and Haselton, M. G. (2008). Changes in women's choice of dress across the ovulatory cycle: Naturalistic and laboratory task-based evidence. *Personality and Social Psychology Bulletin,* 34(11), 1451-1460. doi: 10.1177/0146167208323103

Ellsworth, R. M. (2011). The human that never evolved. *Evol. Psychol.,* 9(3), 325-333.

Emera, D., Romero, R. and Wagner, G. (2012). The evolution of menstruation: A new model for genetic assimilation: Explaining molecular origins of maternal responses to fetal invasiveness. *BioEssays: News and Reviews in Molecular, Cellular and Developmental Biology,* 34(1), 26-35. doi: 10.1002/bies.201100099; 10.1002/bies.201100099.

Euling, S. Y., Herman-Giddens, M. E., Lee, P. A., Selevan, S. G., Juul, A., Sorensen, T. I., Swan, S. H. (2008). Examination of US puberty-timing data from 1940 to 1994 for secular trends: Panel findings. *Pediatrics,* 121 Suppl. 3, S172-91. doi: 10.1542/peds.2007-1813D.

Fessler, D. M. (2003). No time to eat: An adaptationist account of periovulatory behavioral changes. *The Quarterly Review of Biology,* 78 (1), 3-21.

Finn, C. A. (1996). Why do women menstruate? Historical and evolutionary review. *European Journal of Obstetrics, Gynecology, and Reproductive Biology,* 70(1), 3-8.

Finn, C. A. (1998). Menstruation: A nonadaptive consequence of uterine evolution. *The Quarterly Review of Biology,* 73(2), 163-173.

Fisher, M. L. (2004). Female intrasexual competition decreases female facial attractiveness. *Proceedings. Biological Sciences/the Royal Society,* 271 Suppl. 5, S283-5. doi: 10.1098/rsbl.2004.0160

Furtbauer, I., Heistermann, M., Schulke, O., and Ostner, J. (2011). Concealed fertility and extended female sexuality in a non-human primate (macaca assamensis). *PloS One,* 6(8), e23105. doi: 10.1371/journal.pone.0023105

Furtbauer, I., Mundry, R., Heistermann, M., Schulke, O., and Ostner, J. (2011). You mate, I mate: Macaque females synchronize sex not cycles. *PloS One,* 6(10), e26144. doi: 10.1371/journal.pone.0026144.

Gangestad, S. W., Thornhill, R. and Garver-Apgar, C. E. (2005). Adaptations to ovulation. In: D. M. Buss (Ed.), *The handbook of evolutionary psychology* (pp. 344-371). Hoboken, NJ: John Wiley and Sons.

Gangestad, S. W., Thornhill, R. and Garver-Apgar, C. E. (2005). Adaptations to ovulation: Implications for sexual and social behavior. *Current Directions in Psychological Science,* 14, 312-316.

Gangestad, S. W., Simpson, J. A., Cousins, A. J., Garver-Apgar, C. E., and Christensen, P. N. (2004). Women's preferences for male behavioral displays change across the menstrual cycle. *Psychological Science,* 15(3), 203-207.

Gangestad, S. W. and Thornhill, R. (1998). Menstrual cycle variation in women's preferences for the scent of symmetrical men. *Proceedings. Biological Sciences/the Royal Society,* 265(1399), 927-933. doi: 10.1098/rspb.1998.0380

Gangestad, S. W. and Thornhill, R. (2008). Human oestrus. *Proceedings. Biological Sciences/the Royal Society,* 275(1638), 991-1000. doi: 10. 1098/rspb.2007.1425.

Gangestad, S. W., Thornhill, R. and Garver, C. E. (2002). Changes in women's sexual interests and their partners' mate-retention tactics across the menstrual cycle: Evidence for shifting conflicts of interest. *Proceedings. Biological Sciences/the Royal Society,* 269(1494), 975-982. doi: 10. 1098/rspb.2001.1952.

Gangestad, S. W., Thornhill, R. and Garver-Apgar, C. E. (2005). Women's sexual interests across the ovulatory cycle depend on primary partner developmental instability. *Proceedings. Biological Sciences/the Royal Society,* 272(1576), 2023-2027. doi: 10.1098/rspb.2005.3112.

Gellersen, B. and Brosens, J. (2003). Cyclic AMP and progesterone receptor cross-talk in human endometrium: A decidualizing affair. *The Journal of Endocrinology,* 178(3), 357-372.

Gesquiere, L. R., Wango, E. O., Alberts, S. C., and Altmann, J. (2007). Mechanisms of sexual selection: Sexual swellings and estrogen concentrations as fertility indicators and cues for male consort decisions in wild baboons. *Hormones and Behavior,* 51(1), 114-125. doi: 10.1016/j. yhbeh.2006.08.010.

Gilby, I. C., Emery Thompson, M., Ruane, J. D., and Wrangham, R. (2010). No evidence of short-term exchange of meat for sex among chimpanzees. *Journal of Human Evolution,* 59(1), 44-53. doi: 10.1016/j.jhevol. 2010. 02.006.

Gong, T. T., Wu, Q. J., Vogtmann, E., Lin, B., and Wang, Y. L. (2012). Age at menarche and risk of ovarian cancer: A meta-analysis of epidemiological studies. *International Journal of Cancer. Journal International Du Cancer,* doi: 10.1002/ijc.27952; 10.1002/ijc.27952.

Gueguen, N. (2009). The receptivity of women to courtship solicitation across the menstrual cycle: A field experiment. *Biological Psychology,* 80(3), 321-324. doi: 10.1016/j.biopsycho.2008.11.004.

Guillermo, C. J., Manlove, H. A., Gray, P. B., Zava, D. T., and Marrs, C. R. (2010). Female social and sexual interest across the menstrual cycle: The roles of pain, sleep and hormones. *BMC Women's Health,* 10, 19. doi: 10. 1186/1472-6874-10-19.

Hamilton, W. J. (1984). Significance of paternal investment by primates to the evolution of male-female associations. In: D. M. Taub (Ed.), *Primate paternalism* (). New York: Van Nostrand Reinhold Company.

Haselton, M. G. and Gildersleeve, K. (2011). Can men detect ovulation? *Current Directions in Psychological Science,* 20(2), 87-92.

Haselton, M. G. and Miller, G. F. (2006). Evidence for ovulatory shifts in attraction to artistic and entrepreneurial excellence. *Human Nature,* 17, 50-73.

Haselton, M. G. and Gangestad, S. W. (2006). Conditional expression of women's desires and men's mate guarding across the ovulatory cycle. *Hormones and Behavior,* 49(4), 509-518. doi: 10.1016/j.yhbeh.2005. 10. 006.

Haselton, M. G., Mortezaie, M., Pillsworth, E. G., Bleske-Rechek, A., and Frederick, D. A. (2007). Ovulatory shifts in human female ornamentation: Near ovulation, women dress to impress. *Hormones and Behavior,* 51(1), 40-45. doi: 10.1016/j.yhbeh.2006.07.007.

Havlíček, J., Dvořáková, R., Bartoš, L., and Flegr, J. (2006). Non-advertized does not mean concealed: Body odour changes across the human menstrual cycle. *Ethology,* 112(1), 81-90. doi: 10.1111/j.1439-0310. 2006. 01125.x

Heistermann, M., Ziegler, T., van Schaik, C. P., Launhardt, K., Winkler, P., and Hodges, J. K. (2001). Loss of oestrus, concealed ovulation and paternity confusion in free-ranging hanuman langurs. *Proceedings. Biological Sciences/the Royal Society,* 268(1484), 2445-2451. doi: 10. 1098/rspb.2001.1833

Hrdy, S. B. (1979). Infanticide among animals: A review, classification, and examination of the implications for the reproductive strategies of females. *Ethol Sociobiol,* 1, 13-40.

Hrdy, S. B. (1981). *The woman that never evolved.* Cambridge: Harvard University Press.

Imkampe, A. K. and Bates, T. (2012). Correlation of age at oral contraceptive pill start with age at breast cancer diagnosis. *The Breast Journal,* 18(1), 35-40. doi: 10.1111/j.1524-4741.2011.01181.x; 10.1111/j.1524-4741. 2011.01181.x

Johnston, V. S., Hagel, R., Franklin, M., Fink, B., and Grammer, K. (2001). Male facial attractiveness: Evidence for hormone-mediated adaptive design. *Evolution and Human Behavior,* 22(4), 251-267. doi: 10.1016/ S1090-5138(01)00066-6.

Juul, A., Teilmann, G., Scheike, T., Hertel, N. T., Holm, K., Laursen, E. M., Skakkebaek, N. E. (2006). Pubertal development in Danish children: Comparison of recent european and US data. *International Journal of Andrology,* 29(1), 247-55; discussion 286-90. doi: 10.1111/j.1365-2605.2005.00556.x

Kaplowitz, P. B. and Oberfield, S. E. (1999). Reexamination of the age limit for defining when puberty is precocious in girls in the united states: Implications for evaluation and treatment. *Pediatrics,* 104(4 Pt 1), 936-941.

Kirchengast, S. and Gartner, M. (2002). Changes in fat distribution (WHR) and body weight across the menstrual cycle. *Collegium Antropologicum,* 26 Suppl., 47-57.

Krug, R., Moelle, M. and Fehm, H. L. (1999). Variations across the menstrual cycle in EEG activity during thinking and mental relaxation. *Journal of Psychophysiology,* 13, 163-172.

Kuukasiarvi, S., Eriksson, C. J. P., Koskela, E., Mappes, T., Nissinen, K., and Rantala, M. J. (2004). Attractiveness of women's body odors over the menstrual cycle: The role of oral contraceptives and receiver sex. *Behavioral Ecology,* 15, 579-584.

Labied, S., Kajihara, T., Madureira, P. A., Fusi, L., Jones, M. C., Higham, J. M., Brosens, J. J. (2006). Progestins regulate the expression and activity of the forkhead transcription factor FOXO1 in differentiating human endometrium. *Molecular Endocrinology (Baltimore, Md.),* 20(1), 35-44. doi: 10.1210/me.2005-0275.

Lens, I., Driesmans, K., Pandelaere, M., and Janssens, K. (2012). Would male conspicuous consumption capture the female eye? Menstrual cycle effects on women's attention to status products. *Journal of Experimental Social Psychology,* 48(1), 346-349. doi: 10.1016/j.jesp.2011.06.004.

Lockwood, C. J., Krikun, G., Hausknecht, V. A., Papp, C., and Schatz, F. (1998). Matrix metalloproteinase and matrix metalloproteinase inhibitor expression in endometrial stromal cells during progestin-initiated decidualization and menstruation-related progestin withdrawal. *Endocrinology,* 139(11), 4607-4613.

Lu, A., Beehner, J. C., Czekala, N. M., and Borries, C. (2012). Juggling priorities: Female mating tactics in phayre's leaf monkeys. *American Journal of Primatology,* 74(5), 471-481. doi: 10.1002/ajp.22004; 10.1002/ajp.22004.

Macrae, C. N., Alnwick, K. A., Milne, A. B., and Schloerscheidt, A. M. (2002). Person perception across the menstrual cycle: Hormonal influences on social-cognitive functioning. *Psychological Science,* 13(6), 532-536.

Manning, J. T., Scutt, D., Whitehouse, G. H., Leinster, S. J., and Walton, J. M. (1996). Asymmetry and the menstrual cycle in women. *Ethology and Sociobiology,* 17(2), 129-143. doi: 10.1016/0162-3095(96)00001-5.

Marlowe, F. W. (2004). Is human ovulation concealed? Evidence from conception beliefs in a hunter-gatherer society. *Archives of Sexual Behavior,* 33(5), 427-432. doi: 10.1023/B:ASEB.0000037423.84026.1f

Martin, R. D. (2003). Human reproduction: A comparative background for medical hypotheses. *Journal of Reproductive Immunology,* 59(2), 111-135.

Matchock, R. L. and Susman, E. J. (2006). Family composition and menarcheal age: Anti-inbreeding strategies. *American Journal of Human Biology: The Official Journal of the Human Biology Council,* 18(4), 481-491. doi: 10.1002/ajhb.20508.

McClintock, M. K. (1971). Menstrual synchrony and supression. *Nature,* 229, 244-245.

Midyett, L. K., Moore, W. V. and Jacobson, J. D. (2003). Are pubertal changes in girls before age 8 benign? *Pediatrics,* 111(1), 47-51.

Miller, G., Tybur, J. and Jordan, B. D. (2007). Ovulatory cycle effects on tip earnings by lap dancers. *Evol. Hum. Behav.,* 28, 375-381.

Miller, S. L. and Maner, J. K. (2010). Scent of a woman: Men's testosterone responses to olfactory ovulation cues. *Psychological Science,* 21(2), 276-283. doi: 10.1177/0956797609357733.

Miller, S. L. and Maner, J. K. (2011). Ovulation as a male mating prime: Subtle signs of women's fertility influence men's mating cognition and behavior. *Journal of Personality and Social Psychology,* 100(2), 295-308. doi: 10.1037/a0020930.

Nicolson, N. A. (1987). Infants, mothers and other females. In: B. B. Smuts, D. L. Cheney, R. M. Seyfarth, R. W. Wrangham and T. T. Struhsaker (Eds.), *Primate societies* (pp. 330-342). Chicago and London: The University of Chicago Press.

Pawlowski, B. (1999). Loss of oestrus and concealed ovulation in human evolution: The case against the sexual-selection hypothesis. *Current Anthropology,* 40, 257-275.

Penton- Voak, I. S., Perrett, D. I., Castles, D., Burt, M., Kobayashi, T., and Murray, L. K. (1999). Female preference for male faces changes cyclically. *Nature,* 399, 741-742.

Pillsworth, E. G. and Haselton, M. G. (2006). Male sexual attractiveness predicts differential ovulatory shifts in female extra-pair attraction and male mate retention male. *Evol. Hum. Behav.,* 27, 247-324.

Pipitone, R. N. and Gallup, G. G. (2008). Women's voice attractiveness varies across the menstrual cycle. *Evol. Hum. Behav.,* 28, 268-274.

Puts, D. A. (2005). Mating context and menstrual phase affect women's preferences for male voice pitch. *Evolution and Human Behavior,* 26(5), 388-397. doi: 10.1016/j.evolhumbehav.2005.03.001

Rasweiler, J. J., 4th, Badwaik, N. K. and Mechineni, K. V. (2011). Ovulation, fertilization, and early embryonic development in the menstruating fruit bat, carollia perspicillata. *Anatomical Record (Hoboken, N.J.: 2007),* 294 (3), 506-519. doi: 10.1002/ar.21304; 10.1002/ar.21304.

Rasweiler, J. J., 4th and de Bonilla, H. (1992). Menstruation in short-tailed fruit bats (carollia spp.). *Journal of Reproduction and Fertility,* 95(1), 231-248.

Rigon, F., De Sanctis, V., Bernasconi, S., Bianchin, L., Bona, G., Bozzola, M., Perissinotto, E. (2012). Menstrual pattern and menstrual disorders among adolescents: An update of the italian data. *Italian Journal of Pediatrics,* 38, 38-7288-38-38. doi: 10.1186/1824-7288-38-38; 10.1186/1824-7288-38-38.

Roberts, S. C., Havlicek, J., Flegr, J., Hruskova, M., Little, A. C., Jones, B. C., Petrie, M. (2004). Female facial attractiveness increases during the fertile phase of the menstrual cycle. *The Royal Society; Biology Letters,* 270-272. doi: 10.1098/rsbl.2004.0174.

Rupp, H. A. and Wallen, K. (2007). Sex differences in viewing sexual stimuli: An eye-tracking study in men and women. *Hormones and Behavior,* 51(4), 524-533. doi: 10.1016/j.yhbeh.2007.01.008.

Russo, G., Brambilla, P., Della Beffa, F., Ferrario, M., Pitea, M., Mastropietro, T., Chiumello, G. (2012). Early onset of puberty in young girls: An italian cross-sectional study. *Journal of Endocrinological Investigation,* 35(9), 804-808. doi: 10.3275/8062; 10.3275/8062

Ryan, C. and Jethá, C. (2010). *Sex at dawn: How we mate, why we stray, and what it means for modern relationships.* New York: Harper Perennial.

Saxon, L. (2012). *Sex at dusk: Lifting the shiny wrapping from sex at dawn.* Lexington, KY: Createspace Independent Publising Platform.

Short, R. V., Lewis, P. R., Renfree, M. B., and Shaw, G. (1991). Contraceptive effects of extended lactational amenorrhoea: Beyond the bellagio consensus. *Lancet,* 337(8743), 715-717.

Singh, D. and Bronstad, P. M. (2001). Female body odour is a potential cue to ovulation. *The Royal Society,* 797-801.

Sorensen, K., Mouritsen, A., Aksglaede, L., Hagen, C. P., Mogensen, S. S., and Juul, A. (2012). Recent secular trends in pubertal timing: Implications for evaluation and diagnosis of precocious puberty. *Hormone Research in Paediatrics,* 77(3), 137-145. doi: 10.1159/000336325.

Spencer, N. A., McClintock, M. K., Sellergren, S. A., Bullivant, S., Jacob, S., and Mennella, J. A. (2004). Social chemosignals from breastfeeding women increase sexual motivation. *Hormones and Behavior,* 46(3), 362-370. doi: 10.1016/j.yhbeh.2004.06.002

Stern, K. and McClintock, M. K. (1998). Regulation of ovulation by human pheromones. *Nature,* 392(6672), 177-179. doi: 10.1038/32408.

Strassmann, B. (1996). The evolution of endometrial cycles and menstruation. *The Quarterly Review of Biology,* 71(2), 181-220.

Strassmann, B. I. (1981). Sexual selection, paternal care, and concealed ovulation in humans. *Ethology and Sociobiology,* 2(1), 31-40. doi: 10. 1016/0162-3095(81)90020-0.

Strom, J. O., Ingberg, E., Druvefors, E., Theodorsson, A., and Theodorsson, E. (2012). The female menstrual cycle does not influence testosterone concentrations in male partners. *Journal of Negative Results in Biomedicine,* 11, 1. doi: 10.1186/1477-5751-11-1

Symonds, C. S., Gallagher, P., Thompson, J. M., and Young, A. H. (2004). Effects of the menstrual cycle on mood, neurocognitive and neuroendocrine function in healthy premenopausal women. *Psychological Medicine,* 34(1), 93-102.

Takano, M., Lu, Z., Goto, T., Fusi, L., Higham, J., Francis, J., Kim, J. J. (2007). Transcriptional cross talk between the forkhead transcription factor forkhead box O1A and the progesterone receptor coordinates cell cycle regulation and differentiation in human endometrial stromal cells. *Molecular Endocrinology (Baltimore, Md.),* 21(10), 2334-2349. doi: 10. 1210/me.2007-0058

Taub, D. M. (1980). Female choice and mating strategies among wild barbary macaques (macaca sylvanus L.). In: D. G. Lindburg (Ed.), *The macaques: Studies in ecology, behavior, and evolution* (). New York: Van Nostrand Reinhold Company.

Thornhill, R. and Gangestad, S. W. (2008). *The evolutionary biology of human female sexuality*. New York, NY: Oxford University Press.

Thornhill, R., Gangestad, S. W., Miller, R., Scheyd, G., McCullough, J., and Franklin, M. (2003). Major histocompatibility complex genes, symmetry, and body scent attractiveness in men and women. *Behavioral Ecology, 14*(5), 668-678.

Thornhill, R. and Gangestad, S. W. (1999). The scent of symmetry: A human sex pheromone that signals fitness? *Evolution and Human Behavior, 20*(3), 175-201. doi: 10.1016/S1090-5138(99)00005-7.

Turke, P. W. (1984). Effects of ovulatory concealment and synchrony on protohominid mating systems and parental roles. *Ethology and Sociobiology, 5*(1), 33-44. doi: 10.1016/0162-3095(84)90033-5.

Van Schaik, C. P. and Kappeler, P. (1997). Infanticide risk and the evolution of male-female associations in primates. *Proceedings of the Royal Society of London, Series B, 264*, 1687-1694.

Walker, R. S., Hill, K. R., Flinn, M. V., and Ellsworth, R. M. (2011). Evolutionary history of hunter-gatherer marriage practices. *PloS One, 6* (4), e19066. doi: 10.1371/journal.pone.0019066.

Wallen, K. and Zehr, J. L. (2004). Hormones and history: The evolution and development of primate female sexuality. *Journal of Sex Research, 41*(1), 101-112. doi: 10.1080/00224490409552218.

Watts, D. P. (2007). Effects of male group size, parity, and cycle stage on female chimpanzee copulation rates at ngogo, kibale national park, uganda. *Primates; Journal of Primatology, 48*(3), 222-231. doi: 10.1007/s10329-007-0037-2.

Weingarden, H. and Renshaw, K. D. (2012). Early and late perceived pubertal timing as risk factors for anxiety disorders in adult women. *Journal of Psychiatric Research, 46*(11), 1524-1529. doi: 10.1016/j.jpsychires.2012.07.015; 10.1016/j.jpsychires.2012.07.015.

Yoshinaga, K. (2012). Two concepts on the immunological aspect of blastocyst implantation. *The Journal of Reproduction and Development, 58*(2), 196-203.

Zhang, X., Zhu, C., Lin, H., Yang, Q., Ou, Q., Li, Y., Wang, H. (2007). Wild fulvous fruit bats (rousettus leschenaulti) exhibit human-like menstrual cycle. *Biology of Reproduction, 77*(2), 358-364. doi: 10.1095/biolreprod.106.058958.

Zuckerman, S. (1932). The comparative physiology of the menstrual cycle. *British Medical Journal, 2*(3754), 1093-1097.

In: Menstrual Cycle
Editor: Madeleine Gosselin

ISBN: 978-1-62417-945-7
© 2013 Nova Science Publishers, Inc.

Chapter II

Functional and Structural Brain Alterations Associated with Menstrual Pain

Cheng-Hao Tu[1,2]*, David M. Niddam*[1,2,3]
and Jen-Chuen Hsieh[1,2,*]

[1]Institute of Brain Science, National Yang-Ming University,
Taipei, Taiwan
[2]Integrated Brain Research Unit,
Department of Medical Research and Education,
Taipei Veterans General Hospital, Taipei, Taiwan
[3]Brain Research Center, Department of Research and Development,
National Yang-Ming University, Taiwan

Abstract

Dysmenorrhea is a widely presented gynecological disorder for women in the childbearing age. Females with dysmenorrhea suffer from

* Corresponding author: Jen-Chuen Hsieh, MD, PhD. Institute of Brain Science, National Yang-Ming University, Laboratory of Integrated Brain Research, Taipei Veterans General Hospital. No. 201, Sect. 2, Shih-Pai Rd., Taipei 112, Taiwan. E-mail: jchsieh@ym.edu.tw; jchsieh@vghtpe.gov.tw; Tel: (886)-2-28757480, (886)-2-28267906; Fax: (886)-2-28745182.

disabling, cramping pain emanating from the lower abdomen with the onset of menstrual flow and the pain persists for 24–72 hours. Recent studies further disclosed that central sensitization exists in dysmenorrhea as hyperalgesia spans different spinal segments and multiple tissue systems (e.g., skin and muscle) and extends to non-referred pain areas during the menstrual phase. Moreover, menstrual pain is associated with functional and structural alterations in highly specified regions involved in pain transmission and modulation, generation of the affective experience, and regulation of endocrine function. The adaptive and mal-adaptive changes in the brain may be engaged simultaneously and dynamically and that some of these regions may underpin the hyperalgesia in dysmenorrhea.

The functional and structural brain alterations may either be either state-related or trait-related. Where state-related changes are associated with the presence of menstrual pain, trait-related changes exist even in the absence of symptoms.

When comparing pain and pain-free states, the rapid state-related structural changes in several regions correlating with the severity of the menstrual pain experience, suggesting that these changes are primary changes rather than epiphenomena. Some of the observed state-related structural alterations even persisted into the pain-free state indicating an accumulating effect of the cyclic menstrual pain. This notion is supported by a correlation of gray matter volume in these regions with menstrual pain duration.

More specifically, regions involved in pain modulation and affect regulation exhibited hypertrophy and regions associated with pain transmission showed atrophic changes.

Using positron emission topography to study state-related changes in glucose metabolism, the alterations in central processing of menstrual pain suggest that a disinhibitiondisinhibition of a thalamo-orbitofrontal-prefrontal network may promote central sensitization during menstruation. On the other hand, reduced metabolism was also found in sensory-discriminative areas, indicating a down regulation in pain transmission pathways.

These findings are congruent with the structural brain alterations observed in dysmenorrhea. Overall, these results indicate that the adolescent brain is vulnerable to menstrual pain. Considering the high prevalence rate of dysmenorrhea and the early onset of primary dysmenorrhea, these findings mandate a great demand to revisit dysmenorrhea regarding its impact on the brain and other clinical pain conditions. Like the migraine, dysmenorrhea might be considered a chronic disease with episodic features but largely confined to the menstrual phase.

Section I. Introduction

Dysmenorrhea is the most common gynecological disorder for women in the reproductive age. Dysmenorrhea patients suffer from disabling cramping pain emanating from the lower abdomen. It has been estimated that absenteeism due to severe dysmenorrhea may cause about 600 million lost working hours or 2 billion dollars annually in the United States [1]. Clinically, dysmenorrhea can be categorized as *Primary* and *Secondary* [2]. *Primary* dysmenorrhea refers to menstrual pain without macroscopic pelvic abnormality. *Secondary* dysmenorrhea refers to menstrual pain associated with pelvic abnormality (i.e., endometriosis) and occurs less frequently than primary dysmenorrhea [2].

In this chapter, we mainly focus on supraspinal changes associated with dysmenorrhea. FirstInitially, we give a shortshortly review the characteristics of dysmenorrhea and what is known about the pathophysiological mechanisms. Second, we briefly introduce the current understanding of how pain is processed in the brain. We then move on to discuss our findings regarding the impact of dysmenorrhea on the brain. Finally, we discuss the possible implications of these findings and their clinical relevance.

1.1. Clinical Features

Individuals with dysmenorrhea suffer from fluctuating, spasmodic menstrual cramping pain emanating from the suprapubic area. The cramping pain typically starts a few hours before or with onset of the menstrual flow, and last for 24 to 72 hours in primary dysmenorrhea [3]. The menstrual pain may radiate into the inner aspects of the thighs or lumbosacral region. Backache, nausea, vomiting, and diarrhea may also accompany dysmenorrhea [4]. These symptoms may be of such incapacitating severity that absence from school or work is required for days. Typically, primary dysmenorrhea presents with or shortly (within 6 to 12 months) after menarche. Since primary dysmenorrhea only presents in ovulatory cycles, it is less common during early adolescence with anovulatory menstrual cycles [2], and is most prevalent in the early 20'ies [5]. The typical history of suprapubic pain associated with the menstrual flow beginning in adolescence and the absence of any positive findings in the physical examination are key diagnostic features [6]. However, there is no specific laboratory test for primary dysmenorrhea. In contrast, secondary dysmenorrhea is associated with observable pelvic abnormality, it presents at a later stage (years after the manarche), and may persist for a prolonged period of time [3].

1.2. Prevalence

Since the majority of dysmenorrhea in adolescents is *primary* [2], the epidemiology may mainly reflect the prevalence rate of primary dysmenorrhea. In the western society, an investigation in United States including 2,699 menarcheal adolescents (aged 12 to 17 years) revealed that dysmenorrhea was present in 59.7% of the study population, and 14% frequently missed school because of dysmenorrhea [7]. Another study of 1,546 menstruating Canadian women (aged 18 years and above) also found that 60% had dysmenorrhea, and 17% of them reported absenteeism from school or work due to dysmenorrhea [8]. Eighty percent of 388 Australian adolescents (aged 17 to 18 years) also reported experiencing dysmenorrhea and 53% of them reported limitation of activities [9]. Fifty-six percent of 4,992 Italian females (aged 13 to 21 years) report some degree of menstrual pain and 6.2% of these subjects wereare limiting their daily activity by severe dysmenorrhea [10]. In Asia, a large-scale epidemiological study of 5,561 Singaporean female adolescents (aged 12 to 19 years) reported that 83.2% of the subjects experienced dysmenorrhea, and 24% reported school absenteeism owing to it [11]. An investigation in Malaysia among 1,075 menarcheal girls (aged 13 to 19 years) revealed that 74.5% had dysmenorrhea while 21.5% of them considered dysmenorrhea to be a leading reason to miss school [12]. In Japan and Korea, two recent studies included 1,431 Japanese and 538 Korean female adolescents (aged 16 to 18 years in Japan and 14 to 18 years in Korea) showed 85% and 82% of subjects experiencing dysmenorrhea, respectively [13, 14]. The prevalence rate of dysmenorrhea around the world is summarized in Table 1. It is noteworthy to mention that the severity of dysmenorrhea may be influenced by ethnic factors. An early study in the United States reported that the subgroups of African-American and Caucasian adolescents had similar prevalence rates of dysmenorrhea, but the former had nearly double the rate of school absenteeism of due to menstrual pain (African-American: 23.6%, Caucasian: 12.3%) [7]. A study on Hispanic adolescents in the United State reported that the rate of severe menstrual pain was three times higher than the previously mentioned investigation (Hispanic: 42%, African-American and Caucasian: 14%) [7, 15]. In Asia, a recent study on menarcheal girls in

Malaysia reported a significant difference in the prevalence rate of dysmenorrhea among Malayasian (79.7%), Chinese (69.8%), and Indian (82.4%) subgroups [12]. Thus, ethnic factors need to be considered in the study of dysmenorrhea.

Table 1. Studies of Prevalence Rate of Dysmenorrhea in Different Countries

Author	Pub. year	Sample size	Age	Prevalence	Country
Grandi et al. [115]	2012	408	19-25	81.4%	Italy
Gumanga and Kwame-Aryee [116]	2012	456	14-19	74.4%	Ghana
Karuot et al. [117]	2012	352	18-26	38.1%	Lebanon
Kitamura et al. [13]	2012	1431	16-18	85%	Japan
Rigon et al. [10]	2012	4992	13-21	56%	Italy
Santina et al. [118]	2012	389	13-19	74.3%	Lebanon
Lee et al. [14]	2011	538	14-18	82%	Korea
Muhammad et al. [119]	2011	900	18-59	55.3%	Egypt
Omidvar and Begum [120]	2011	194	18-27	78.2%	India
Tavallaee et al. [121]	2011	381	16-56	90%	Iran
Wong [122]	2011	1295	13-19	76%	Malaysia
Agarwal and Agarwal [123]	2010	970	15-20	79.67%	India
Al-Kindi and Al-Bulushi [124]	2010	404	15-23	94%	Oman
Eryilmaz et al. [125]	2010	1951	13-18	68.1-72.2%	Turkey
Ortiz [126]	2010	1539	17-35	62.4%	Mexico
Parker et al. [127]	2010	1051	15-19	93.0%	Australia
Wong and Khoo [12]	2010	1092	13-19	74.5%	Malaysia
Unsal et al. [128]	2010	623	17-30	72.7%	Turkey
Agarwal and Venkat [11]	2009	5561	12-19	83.2%	Singapore
Chan et al. [129]	2009	5609	13-18	68.7%	Hong Kong
Fawole et al. [130]	2009	1213	9-23	72.7%	Nigeria
Yamamoto et al. [131]	2009	221	18-25	79.0%	Japan
Zegeye et al. [132]	2009	612	14-19	72.0%	Ethiopia
Pitts et al. [133]	2008	1983	16-49	71.7%	Australian

Table 1. (Continued)

Author	Pub. year	Sample size	Age	Prevalence	Country
Sharma et al. [134]	2008	198	13-19	67.2%	India
Ortiz et al. [135]	2007	285	17-33	67.0%	Mexico
Banikarim et al. [15]	2000	706	15-18	85.0%	United States
Hillen et al. [9]	1999	384	15-17	80.0%	Australia
Gürel and Gürel [136]	1998	235	18-56	57.0%	Turkey
Harlow and Park [137]	1996	165	17-19	71.6%	United States
Jamieson and Steege [138]	1996	533	18-45	90.0%	United States
Ng et al. [139]	1992	415	15-54	51.3%	Singapore
Sundell et al. [140]	1990	489	24	67.0%	Sweden
Thomas et al. [141]	1990	768	15-34	72.3%	Nigeria
Pullon et al. [142]	1988	1826	16-54	53.0%	New Zealand
Andersch and Milsom [143]	1982	596	19	72.4%	Sweden
Klein and Litt [7]	1981	2699	12-17	59.7%	United States

Note: These studies were found by searching PubMed using "dysmenorrhea" and "prevalence" as keywords at the end of September, 2012. The search resulted in 561 studies. We excluded intervention studies, studies which did not report the prevalence rate of dysmenorrhea, and review articles. Thirty-seven studies were left and listed in the table. Studies are sorted chronologically and then in alphabetical order of author's name.

1.3. Comorbidities

Clinically, dysmenorrhea is often comorbid with other idiopathic pain disorders. Irritable bowel syndrome (IBS) and fibromyalgia are two pain conditions with central sensitization [16, 17] that have a higher prevalence rate in females [18, 19] and are often comorbid with dysmenorrhea [20]. Furthermore, IBS patients have more severe clinical symptoms with concomitant dysmenorrhea than with IBS alone [21], and the treatment of dysmenorrhea can improve the symptoms of IBS [22].

A recent study further suggests that menstrual pain is associated with the possibility of having premenstrual dysphoric disorder [23], the most severe form of premenstrual symptoms. Finally, there are also indications that primary dysmenorrhea is associated with elevated state anxiety levels during menstruation [24, 25].

1.4. Pathophysiology

The etiology of primary dysmenorrhea has not been fully elucidated. The local inflammatory environment of the menstruating uterus has been suggested as the primary mechanism, but sensitization in the central nervous system may also play a role [3]. Peripherally, primary dysmenorrhea has been suggested to be a sex-hormone related disorder accompanied by a decrease of progesterone before menstruation [2]. The decline of uterine progesterone levels in the late luteal phase results in an increase of arachidonic acid, which is subsequently metabolized into eicosanoids (including leukotrienes [LT] and prostaglandins [PG]).

It has been shown that dysmenorrhic women receiving no medication had four times higher endometrial PGF2-α levels than the eumenorrheic women on the first day of the menstrual period [26]. The level of PGF2-α was directly proportional to the intensity of menstrual pain and symptoms of dysmenorrhea [4]. Moreover, primary dysmenorrhea is associated with higher concentrations of menstrual LT-C4/D4 [27]. Since LT-C4 has binding sites in myometrial cells [28], it is possible that LT contribute to uterine hypercontractility.

Indeed, primary dysmenorrhea patients have higher basal uterine tone, active pressures, and increased number of uterine contractions compared to normal women [4]. Thus, the cascade response of PG and LT, which mediate hyperalgesia and inflammatory responses, may cause vasoconstriction, ischemia and myometrial contraction [3].

In addition to peripheral mechanisms, sensitization in the central nervous system may also play a role in dysmenorrhea. Using electric stimulation, it has been demonstrated that hyperalgesia exist in deep tissue (i.e., subcutaneous and muscle) at both referred and non-referred pain sites throughout the menstrual cycle in dysmenorrhea patients [29].

Furthermore, during the menstrual period hyperalgesia extends to the skin as tested with thermal and pressure stimulation but not tactile stimulation [30].

In a laser-evoked potential study, dysmenorrhea patients revealed longer latencies of pain-evoked potentials and a higher magnitude of supra-threshold pain stimulation compared to healthy subjects [24]. The aforementioned studies indicate an enhanced pain perception in patients with dysmenorrhea, possibly as a result of both peripheral and central sensitization.

1.5. Chronification of Pain

Prolonged nociceptive input from the periphery to the central nervous system can induce functional and structural alterations throughout the nervous system and is known to result in central sensitization [31].

Initially, peripheral and central sensitization act together to induce spontaneous ongoing pain, enhanced pain sensitivity (hyperalgesia), a lowered pain threshold turning non-nociceptive input into pain (allodynia), and referred pain. With further pain chronification, pathological changes at peripheral, spinal and supraspinal levels take place. Some of these changes may become independent of the peripheral input and even persist in their absence.

At the supraspinal level, brain imaging studies have shown that chronic pain may induce changes in brain chemistry [32, 33], brain processing [34-37], and in macroscopic brain structures [38].

Clinical pain states of heterogeneous etiology have been associated with abnormal cognitive/ emotional and sensory processing albeit with subtle differences between clinical states [34]. Because chronic pain is a heterogeneous group of conditions arising from variousvaries tissue systems, the different types cannot be expected to result in identical brain alterations. Factors such as cyclicity, pain history, pain distribution, cause of pain, and psychological setup varies across individuals as well as studies. Chronic pain is discomforting and distressing for most individuals and is highly comorbid with mood and anxiety disorders [39]. Psychiatric comorbidity may further result in separate central changes and in a specific brain "signature".

Section II. Structural and Functional Alterations in the Brain of Dysmenorrhea Patients

In the past two decades, non-invasive functional brain imaging techniques have greatly increased our knowledge of pain processing in the brain. It is now well-accepted that noxious information is processed by a widely distributed, hierarchically-interconnected neural network, commonly referred to as the "pain matrix", in the brain [40, 41]. The majority of functional brain imaging studies, mainly conducted using positron emission tomography (PET) and functional magnetic resonance imaging (fMRI), examined the brain processing in response to painful cutaneous stimulation.

The most commonly found brain regions responding to cutaneous pain stimuli include primary somatosensory cortex (SI), secondary somatosensory cortex (SII), anterior cingulate cortex (ACC), insula, and thalamus. Other less consistently engaged regions include the prefrontal cortex (PFC), premotor and motor cortex, and cerebellum [34, 37, 42].

Other regions such as the basal ganglia, amygdala, hippocampus, and parietal and temporal cortices may also be engaged depending on the particular pain condition or comparison [37]. The neuroanatomical regions involved in pain processing have simplistically been categorized as belonging to the sensory-discriminatory related "lateral pain system" and/ or the affective-cognitive related "medial pain system" [43].

An additional component of pain processing may involve a motor component such as in, e.g., motor-defensive or reorienting responses. Evidences suggests that the SI, SII, and posterior insula are associated with the sensory-discriminative aspects of pain processing while ACC, anterior insula and PFC are associated with affective-cognitive aspects of pain processing [34, 44-46].

However, because the role of different brain regions are more or less dependenting upon the interplay of factors influencing pain perception, the categorization is not always consistent regarding the function of particular regions, especially when concerned with higher-order pain processing areas. It is important to emphasize that although acute cutaneous pain shares many commonalities in brain processing with acute muscle pain [47], substantial differences exist when compared to acute visceral pain.

2.1. Visceral Pain Processing in the Brain

The cumulating literature on brain processing of visceral pain has revealed overlapping but also distinct brain networks processing visceral and cutaneous pain. The different brain activation patterns between the two types of pain may partially be attributed to the separate afferent pathways.

Cutaneous nociceptive input are transmitted to the brain via the lateral spinothalamic tract (STT) while nociceptive input from visceral organs are transmitted not only via the lateral STT but also via multiple other pathways including the vagal, glossopharyngeal, and cranial nerves and the spinal dorsal column (DC) [48-51].

An early meta-analysis of visceral brain imaging studies revealed that the most consistently activated regions were the anterior insula and ACC [35]. The PFC, orbitofrontal cortex (OFC), motor cortex, SI, SII, thalamus, and inferior parietal cortex were less commonly reported. The least consistently reported regions were the subcortical regions such as amygdala, periaqueductal gray matter (PAG), lentiform nucleus, and caudate nucleus [35, 48, 52].

These activation patterns may partially explain the clinical observations that somatic sensation is well localized while localization of visceral sensation is dull and poorly localized [48]. It is noteworthy to mention that the activation maps of visceral pain are inconsistent across different visceral disease entities and stimulation sites.

Apparently, different parts of the gastrointestinal tract may preferentially engage different brain regions. Visceral stimulation using rectal distension in both healthy subjects and in patients with irritable bowel syndrome (IBS) results in a more pronounced activation in the medial pain system (i.e., PFC, OFC, and rostral ACC) and less in the lateral pain system (i.e., SI and SII) [35, 53-56]. In contrast, esophageal stimulation more frequently engage sensorimotor regions, including SI and SII, and dorsal ACC [52, 57-60].

Recent studies using painful proximal gastric distension in both healthy subjects and in functional dyspepsia patients reported significant activation in SI/SII areas [61-63], while earlier studies in healthy subjects stimulating the gastric fundus and antrum failed to engage SI/SII [48, 64].

Thus, it is likely that visceral pain originating from different organs may result in different activation patterns of the brain. Some of the important regions and pathways found to be involved in visceral pain processing are illustrated in Figure 1A.

2.2. Structural Brain Alterations in Dysmenorrhea

2.2.1. Gray Matter Alterations in Chronic Pain

Structural alterations in the grey matter (GM) of the brain can be studied by segmentation of high-resolution anatomical MRI scans. Convergent studies have demonstrated that chronic sustained pain of various etiologies is accompanied by GM alterations in the brain.

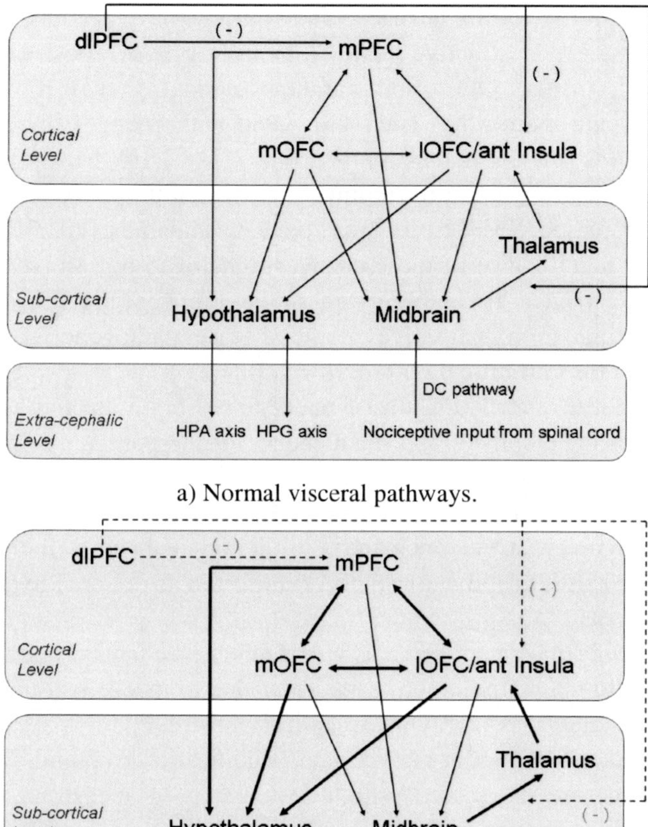

a) Normal visceral pathways.

b) Dysregulaalted pathways in dysmenorrheal.

Figure 1. Diagram of the normal and dysregulated visceral pain pathways. (A) In women without dysmenorrhea, the visceral pain networks are regulated by the dorsolateral prefrontal cortex (dlPFC). The visceral pain network includes the spinal dorsal column (DC), midbrain, thalamus, lateral orbitofrontal cortex (lOFC)/ anterior insula (ant insula), medial orbitofrontal cortex (mOFC), medial prefrontal cortex (mPFC), and hypothalamus. Hypothalamus is the initial point of the hypothalamic-pituitary-adrenal (HPA) and hypothalamic-pituitary-gonadal (HPG) axis. (B) After long-term suffering from dysmenorrhea, changes in dlPFC may result in a dysregulated visceral pain network. "(-)" denotes inhibitory input. Bold line and dashed line denote enhanced and dysfunctioned pathways, respectively.

It has been reported that headache and migraine have been associated with GM atrophy mainly in affective related regions (e.g. ACC, posterior cingulate cortex [PCC], insula, OFC, and parahippocampal gyrus) [65-67], while chronic back pain mainly has been associated with changes in sensorimotor regions (e.g. PFC, SI, and thalamus) [68, 69].

In patients with IBS, cortical thinning has been found in ACC and anterior insula and decreased GM density was found in thalamus [70, 71]. Although the functional significance of these changes remains to be resolved, structural brain alterations have been suggested to be the consequence of ongoing nociceptive stimulation, causative to the disease pathogenesis, and/ or an integral part of the chronification process [72].

This has led to the notion thatof maladaptive brain atrophy that may be responsible for development and maintenance of the pain state. In context of chronic pain, maladaptive plasticity in response to protracted nociceptive input may result in decreased inhibition or increased facilitation.

On the contrary, acute nociceptive infliction in healthy individuals has been associated with adaptive plasticity, manifested as regional hypertrophy in pain-related areas [73].

Adaptive plasticity may serve as a protective mechanism against ongoing input in order to maintain homeostasis. Thus, due to its cyclical nature of pain and pain-free states, it is highly possible that menstrual pain is associated with both state- and trait-related structural abnormalities in the brain. Where state-related changes are associated with the presence of menstrual pain, trait-related changes exist even in the absence of symptoms.

2.2.2. White Matter Alterations in Chronic Pain

The integrity of white matter (WM) tracts can be studied using diffusion tensor imaging (DTI). The DTI measures the diffusion of water in different directions and provides information about the microstructure of WM tracts.

The fractional anisotropy (FA), which calculated from DTI, can be used as an index to further quantify the directional level of WM tracts.

Abnormal FA values have been found in pain-related brain regions and pathways in various chronic pain conditions. In fibromyalgia patients, the thalamus, insula, and thalamocortical tracts revealed decreased FA values while SI, PFC, amygdala, and hippocampus revealed increase FA values compared to normal controls [74]. The neuropathic pain patients also revealed WM changes in OFC, PFC, and posterior parietal cortex regions [75].

Moreover, the patient with IBS revealed increase FA values near insula. The clinical characteristics of IBS (e.g, pain severity, pain unpleasantness, and

IBS duration) further correlated with the FA values near different subregions of insula [76]. Thus, like the GM alterations in brain in chronic pain, the WM in the brain may also be altered after long-term pain suffering.

2.2.3. State- and Trait-Related Grey Matter Alterations in Dysmenorrhea

In our studies [20 and unpublished observation], we addressed possible rapid state-related and long-term trait-related structural alterations of the brain in dysmenorrhea. During the pain-free state, dysmenorrhea patients disclosed trait-related atrophic GM changes in regions involved in pain transmission, higher level sensory processing, and affect regulation, namely medial PFC (mPFC), right central and ventral portions of precuneus, bilateral SII/ posterior insula, right superior tempral gyrus (STG)/mid insula, right culmen, and left cerebellar tonsil. Trait-related hypertrophic GM alterations were found in regions involved in pain modulation and in regulation of the endocrine function, namely right posterior hippocampus/ parahippocampus, ACC/dorsal PCC (dPCC), dorsal midbrain (PAG), hypothalamus, left ventral portion of precuneus, left STG/middle temporal gyrus (MTG), and right cerebellar tonsil. Moreover, trait-related GM changes in key regions involved in top-down pain modulation and in generation of negative affect were related to clinical symptoms.

The right mPFC, bilateral dorsolateral PFC (dlPFC), right premotor cortex, and right lateral OFC (lOFC)/anterior insula were negatively while the right ACC/dPCC and bilateral medial OFC (mOFC) were positively correlated with the menstrual pain experience (i.e., total scores of pain rating index in the McGill Pain Questionnaire [MPQ]). Considering the early onset of dysmenorrhea, these results suggest vulnerability of the adolescent brain to long-term menstrual pain suffering.

Several of the regions exhibiting trait-related alterations also exhibited state-related changes (i.e. between pain and pain-free state) in dysmenorrhea patients (Figure 2). Greater state-related hypertrophic changes were observed in mOFC, right central portion of precuneus, and right hypothalamus while greater atrophic changes were found in SII and ACC/dPCC in dysmenorrhea than control. Moreover, in dysmenorrhea subjects the GM volume differences within hypothalamus and thalamus were significantly positively and negatively correlated with the current menstrual pain experience scores, respectively. These findings suggest that spontaneous recurrent pain results in rapid state-related changes in macroscopic brain structures, and that adaptive and mal-adaptive changes may be engaged simultaneously and dynamically.

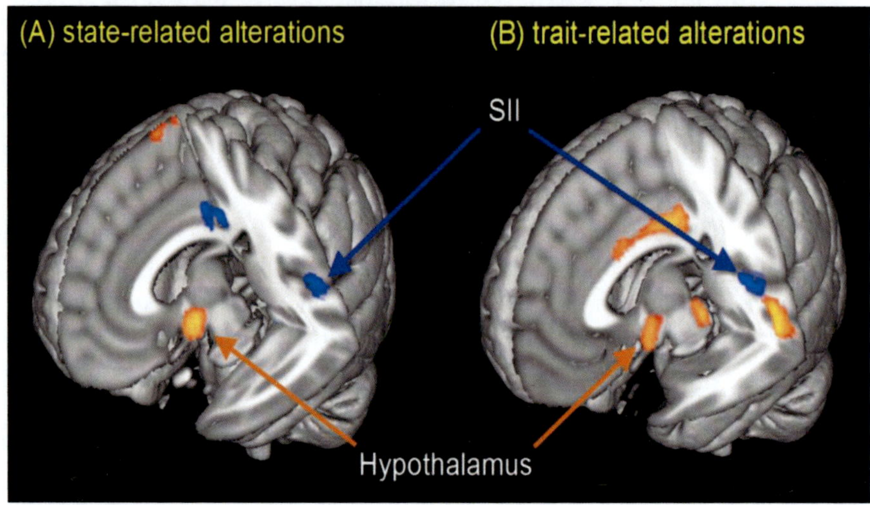

Figure 2. State- and trait-related brain gray matter volume changes in dysmenorrhea patients. Both (A) state-related (during menstrual pain period) and (B) trait-related (during pain-free period) gray matter volume analysis revealed hypertrophic and atrophic changes in hypothalamus and secondary somatosensory area (SII), respectively. The regions are threshold with uncorrected voxel p<0.005 and a cluster extension larger than 150 voxels. The warm colors represent increased volume while cold colors represent decreased volume.

2.2.4. State-and Trait-Related White Matter Alterations in Dysmenorrhea

Long-term suffering from dysmenorrhea may not only alter regional GM volumes but also the local WM tracts in the brain. Using FA as an index, dysmenorrhea patients exhibited trait-related WM tract alterations in pain transmission and modulation pathways. Decreased FA values were found in the corticospinal tract near SI and in the anterior thalamic radiations near the superior frontal gyrus. The corticospinal tract is a descending projection from the cortex to the spinal cord [77], which is functionally associated with the control of sensory afferent input and supports the voluntary execution of skilled movements [78]. The WM alterations in the corticospinal tract may therefore represent an abnormal structural change in the sensory feed-forward loop to the spinal dorsal horn that potentially could contribute in part to the central sensitization known to exist in dysmenorrhea [29, 30]. The anterior thalamic radiation reciprocally connects the anterior and medial regions of the thalamus with the prefrontal cortex [79]. The prefrontal cortex is considered a

3.1. Central Sensitization

Previous studies indicate that central sensitization exists in patients with dysmenorrhea [24, 29, 30]. One plausible contributing mechanism may involve disinhibition of key brain circuits by dlPFC, a region involved in top-down pain modulation [84] (Figure 1B). In dysmenorrhea patients, we observed hypo-metabolism in dlPFC during menstrual pain and a negative correlation between GM volumes in dlPFC and the menstrual pain experience [20, 25]. Together, these findings point to a dysfunctional dlPFC that is further negatively influenced by pain severity. A dysfunctional dlPFC has previously been implicated in disinhibition of orbitofrontal networks, including mPFC and ACC, which may lead to enhanced negative affect [69, 84]. Congruent with this, we also found hyper-metabolism during menstrual pain in mOFC and a positive correlation between GM volumes in mOFC and the menstrual pain experience, while atrophic trait-related GM changes were found in mPFC, which negatively correlated with the menstrual pain experience [20, 25].

A dysfunctional dlPFC may also implicate a dis-inhibited visceral afferent pathway. The dlPFC may influence pain transmission between the midbrain and thalamus and at the level of the anterior insula resulting in the modulation of pain intensity and affect, respectively [84](Figure 1B). In animals, visceral nociceptive afferents are known to project to the ventral- posterior portion of the thalamus via the DC pathway in the spinal cord [51, 85, 86], and then project to the visceral sensory areas in the lateral posterior OFC/ anterior insula [87, 88] (Figure 1B). The DC pathway is considered part of a facilitatory loop that can intensify noxious visceral responses and may be necessary for the maintenance of sensitization associated with chronic visceral pain [89, 90]. The pulvinar, a nucleus located in the posterior portion of the thalamus, has been implicated in a relay of somatosensory information and in directed attention towards sensory stimuli [91]. Furthermore, the lOFC of the right hemisphere has preponderantly been associated with evaluation of aversive stimuli and regulation of negative emotion [92]. Hence, our results suggest a disinhibition of a thalamo-orbitofrontal-prefrontal network that may promote central sensitization in dysmenorrhea in both functional and structural aspects.

Other possible mechanisms that may contribute to maintaining central sensitization involves the hypothalamus. The hypothalamus has the potential to influence menstrual pain through interacting pathways in which it has a decisive role (Figure 1B). The hypothalamus is part of a feedback loop in the hypothalamic-pituitary-gonadal axis which regulates the menstrual cycle. In this loop, the hypothalamus responds to elevated estrogen levels and regulates uterine PG synthesis [93]. An abnormally elevated estrogen level has been found in the late luteal phase in women with primary dysmenorrhea [94], and higher endometrial PGF2-α levels havehas been found in dysmenorrheic women than in eumenorrheic women on the first day of the menstrual period [26]. Moreover, the level of PGF2-α was directly proportional to the menstrual pain intensity and symptoms of dysmenorrhea [4]. Thus, a periodic increased estrogen assault on the hypothalamus may take place which could result in longer-lasting reactive structural GM changes.

Hypothalamus is also a key component of the spino-bulbo-spinal loop, a pain modulatory pathway that may lead to enhanced negative affect and pain amplification [95 76](Figure 1B). Another key region in this loop is the PAG which is well-known for its role in pain modulation. Both of these regions revealed trait-related structural alterations in our study [20]. Other regions providing cortical feedback to this loop include hippocampus and ACC. These two regions also exhibited trait-related hypertrophic changes [20]. The ACC/dPCC is a region consistently associated with pain responses in chronic pain patients [45] and alterations in the hippocampus and amygdala have been reported in animal models of chronic neuropathic pain [96]. In conjunction with the aforementioned dis-inhibited thalamo-orbitofrontal-prefrontal network, the spino-bulbo-spinal loop may play a down-stream role to the central sensitization phenomena since anatomically hypothalamus and PAG receives afferent projections from the mPFC and mOFC [97]. These medial structures could reflect mal-adaptive plasticity underpinning the hyperalgesia known to exist in dysmenorrhea patients.

3.2. Adolescent Health, Pre-Disposition and Comorbidities

Considering that the dysmenorrhea populations in our studies were relatively young and had suffered from regular menstrual pain since adolescence, brain maturation most likely was in progress concomitant with the onset of dysmenorrhea. Since brain maturation is ongoing in adolescents and is more stable in adults [98, 99], our results may not only indicate that the adolescent brain is vulnerable to reoccurring menstrual pain but also that this vulnerability affects the brain at a later stage in adulthood.

Emotional and physiological stress are integral components of dysmenorrhea and two key factors profoundly influencing the brain. Dysmenorrhea has been associated with increased perceived stress levels and the menstrual pain is thought to be aggravated by emotional stress [100]. The hypothalamus, which we found to be enlarged in dysmenorrhea, is also involved in shaping of the physiological stress response through the hypothalamic-pituitary-adrenal (HPA) axis (Figure 1B). Cortisol, a stress indicator secreted from the adrenal cortex into circulation, has been found to vary across the menstrual cycle in women with dysmenorrhea with the highest level during the menstrual phase [101]. Another study found a decreased level of cortisol in dysmenorrhea when collapsing data across the menstrual cycle and a negative correlation of mean cortisol with the duration of dysmenorrhea [102]. However, these findings possibly represent stimulated cortisol and indicate increasingly abnormal stress regulation in face of stimulated stress. One plausible mechanism of HPA dysregulation involves abnormal hippocampal feedback to the hypothalamus since ongoing stress impairs the negative feedback mechanism from the hippocampus to the HPA axis [103]. Congruent with this, trait-related hippocampal hypertrophy was found in our study [20].

The adolescent brain is functionally and structurally sensitive to stress as evidenced by the literature concerned with early-life trauma [104-106]. The sensitivity most likely depends on several factors including stress type, duration, and age of onset. In animal models using adolescent rodents (e.g., 30 to 60 days), chronic stress altered corticolimbic structures, e.g. the hippocampus, amygdala, and prefrontal cortex [107], involved in the modulation of the HPA axis. Furthermore, the recovery period of dendritic morphological changes in prefrontal regions after chronic stress is longer in adolescents than in adulthood [108, 109]. It is therefore possible that repeated stress may have a cumulative effect on stress-induced structural plasticity [110]. Thus, cyclic recurrent menstrual pain has the potential to greatly influence brain development in adolescence.

Taking the above into account, it is possible that menstrual pain may act as a pre-disposing factor for other clinical conditions. It has previously been proposed that dysmenorrhea may act as a precursor stage in women who progress to chronic pelvic pain, since dysmenorrhea often is reported prior to the development of chronic pelvic pain [111]. Premenstrual dysphoric disorder has also been associated with dysmenorrhea and the occurrence of premenstrual dysphoric disorder significantly correlated with the severity of menstrual pain [23, 112]. Other pain conditions that are more prevalent in females [18, 19] and are often comorbid with dysmenorrhea [20] include IBS and fibromyalgia. Indications of enhanced stress responsiveness and a dysregulated HPA axis exist in IBS patients [113, 114]. Interestingly, like in our studies, the hypothalamus was also found to be enlarged in IBS patients [70]. Also, abnormal hippocampal glutamatergic neurotransmission has been found in IBS patients suggesting altered HPA feedback [33]. Taken together, it is conceivable that the early onset of dysmenorrhea may result in a mal-adaptive effect that predisposes to other clinical conditions. Repeated state-related brain alterations induced by menstrual pain in adolescence may result in a cumulative effect that contributes to the aforementioned pre-disposition effect and to the chronification of other clinical pain conditions.

Conclusion

Dysmenorrhea is a widely presented gynecological disorder for women in the childbearing age. It is often comorbid with other idiopathic pain conditions. In a series of studies, we demonstrated that trait- and state-related brain alterations, both functionally and structurally, exist in dysmenorrhea. Overall these alterations included regions involved in top-down pain modulation, affective regulation, and pain transmission. Our studies suggest that adaptive and mal-adaptive changes in the brain may be engaged simultaneously and dynamically in dysmenorrhea. These changes may further provide a possible mechanism for cyclic recurrent menstrual pain to pre-dispose or contribute to the chronification of other clinical pain conditions. Like the migraine, primary dysmenorrhea should be considered a chronic disease with episodic features but largely confined to the menstrual phase. A serious revisit of primary dysmenorrhea regarding its impact on the brain and long-term clinical consequences is needed.

References

[1]	Dawood, M. Y. (1988). Nonsteroidal anti-inflammatory drugs and changing attitudes toward dysmenorrhea. *Am. J. Med.*, 84(5A), 23-9.

[2]	Harel, Z. (2002). A contemporary approach to dysmenorrhea in adolescents. *Paediatr. Drugs*, 4(12), 797-805.

[3]	Tu, F. (2007). Dysmenorrhea: Contemporary Perspectives. *Pain: Clinical Update,* 15 (8).

[4]	Dawood, M. Y. (2006). Primary dysmenorrhea: advances in pathogenesis and management. *Obstet. Gynecol.*, 108(2), 428-41.

[5] Weissman, A. M., Hartz, A. J., Hansen, M. D., Johnson, S. R. (2004). The natural history of primary dysmenorrhoea: a longitudinal study. *BJOG*, 111(4), 345-52.

[6] French, L. (2005). Dysmenorrhea. *Am. Fam. Physician*, 71(2), 285-91.

[7] Klein, J. R., Litt, I. F. (1981). Epidemiology of adolescent dysmenorrhea. *Pediatrics*, 68 (5), 661-4.

[8] Burnett, M. A., Antao, V., Black, A., Feldman, K., Grenville, A., Lea, R., et al. (2005). Prevalence of primary dysmenorrhea in Canada. *J. Obstet. Gynaecol. Can.*, 27(8), 765-70.

[9] Hillen, T. I., Grbavac, S. L., Johnston, P. J., Straton, J. A., Keogh, J. M. (1999). Primary dysmenorrhea in young Western Australian women: prevalence, impact, and knowledge of treatment. *J. Adolesc. Health*, 25(1), 40-5.

[10] Rigon, F., De Sanctis, V., Bernasconi, S., Bianchin, L., Bona, G., Bozzola, M., et al. (2012). Menstrual pattern and menstrual disorders among adolescents: an update of the Italian data. *Ital. J. Pediatr.*, 38, 38.

[11] Agarwal, A., Venkat, A. (2009). Questionnaire study on menstrual disorders in adolescent girls in Singapore. *J. Pediatr. Adolesc. Gynecol.*, 22(6), 365-71.

[12] Wong, L. P., Khoo, E. M. (2010). Dysmenorrhea in a multi-ethnic population of adolescent Asian girls. *Int. J. Gynaecol. Obstet.*, 108(2), 139-42.

[13] Kitamura, M., Takeda, T., Koga, S., Nagase, S., Yaegashi, N. (2012). Relationship between premenstrual symptoms and dysmenorrhea in Japanese high school students. *Arch. Women's Ment. Health*, 15(2), 131-3.

[14] Lee, J. C., Yu, B. K., Byeon, J. H., Lee, K. H., Min, J. H., Park, S. H. (2011). A study on the menstruation of Korean adolescent girls in Seoul. *Korean J. Pediatr.*, 54(5), 201-6.

[15] Banikarim, C., Chacko, M. R., Kelder, S. H. (2000). Prevalence and impact of dysmenorrhea on Hispanic female adolescents. *Arch. Pediatr. Adolesc. Med.*, 154(12), 1226-9.

[16] Wilder-Smith, C. H., Robert-Yap, J. (2007). Abnormal endogenous pain modulation and somatic and visceral hypersensitivity in female patients with irritable bowel syndrome. *World J. Gastroenterol.*, 13(27), 3699-704.

[17] Blumenstiel, K., Gerhardt, A., Rolke, R., Bieber, C., Tesarz, J., Friederich, H. C., et al. (2011). Quantitative sensory testing profiles in

chronic back pain are distinct from those in fibromyalgia. *Clin. J. Pain,* 27(8), 682-90.

[18] Sauer, K., Kemper, C., Glaeske, G. (2011). Fibromyalgia syndrome: prevalence, pharmacological and non-pharmacological interventions in outpatient health care. An analysis of statutory health insurance data. *Joint Bone Spine,* 78(1), 80-4.

[19] Chang, F. Y., Lu, C. L., Chen, T. S. (2010). The current prevalence of irritable bowel syndrome in Asia. *J. Neurogastroenterol. Motil.,* 16(4), 389-400.

[20] Tu, C. H., Niddam, D. M., Chao, H. T., Chen, L. F., Chen, Y. S., Wu, Y. T., et al. (2010). Brain morphological changes associated with cyclic menstrual pain. *Pain,* 150 (3), 462-8.

[21] Altman, G., Cain, K. C., Motzer, S., Jarrett, M., Burr, R., Heitkemper, M. (2006). Increased symptoms in female IBS patients with dysmenorrhea and PMS. *Gastroenterol. Nurs.,* 29(1), 4-11.

[22] Giamberardino, M. A., Costantini, R., Affaitati, G., Fabrizio, A., Lapenna, D., Tafuri, E., et al. (2010). Viscero-visceral hyperalgesia: characterization in different clinical models. *Pain,* 151(2), 307-22.

[23] Issa, B. A., Yussuf, A. D., Olatinwo, A. W., Ighodalo, M. (2010). Premenstrual dysphoric disorder among medical students of a Nigerian university. *Ann. Afr. Med.,* 9 (3), 118-22.

[24] Granot, M., Yarnitsky, D., Itskovitz-Eldor, J., Granovsky, Y., Peer, E., Zimmer, E. Z. (2001). Pain perception in women with dysmenorrhea. *Obstet. Gynecol.,* 98(3), 407-11.

[25] Tu, C. H., Niddam, D. M., Chao, H. T., Liu, R. S., Hwang, R. J., Yeh, T. C., et al. (2009). Abnormal cerebral metabolism during menstrual pain in primary dysmenorrhea. *Neuroimage,* 47(1), 28-35.

[26] Lundstrom, V., Green, K. (1978). Endogenous levels of prostaglandin F2alpha and its main metabolites in plasma and endometrium of normal and dysmenorrheic women. *Am. J. Obstet. Gynecol.,* 130(6), 640-6.

[27] Nigam, S., Benedetto, C., Zonca, M., Leo-Rossberg, I., Lubbert, H., Hammerstein, J. (1991). Increased concentrations of eicosanoids and platelet-activating factor in menstrual blood from women with primary dysmenorrhea. *Eicosanoids,* 4(3), 137-41.

[28] Mitchell, M. D., Grzyboski, C. F. (1987). Arachidonic acid metabolism by lipoxygenase pathways in intrauterine tissues of women at term of pregnancy. *Prostaglandins Leukot. Med.,* 28(3), 303-12.

[29] Giamberardino, M. A., Berkley, K. J., Iezzi, S., de Bigontina, P., Vecchiet, L. (1997). Pain threshold variations in somatic wall tissues as

a function of menstrual cycle, segmental site and tissue depth in non-dysmenorrheic women, dysmenorrheic women and men. *Pain*, 71(2), 187-97.

[30] Bajaj, P., Madsen, H., Arendt-Nielsen, L. (2002). A comparison of modality-specific somatosensory changes during menstruation in dysmenorrheic and nondysmenorrheic women. *Clin. J. Pain*, 18(3), 180-90.

[31] Latremoliere, A., Woolf, C. J. (2009). Central sensitization: a generator of pain hypersensitivity by central neural plasticity. *J. Pain*, 10(9), 895-926.

[32] Grachev, I. D., Fredrickson, B. E., Apkarian, A. V. (2002). Brain chemistry reflects dual states of pain and anxiety in chronic low back pain. *J. Neural. Transm.*, 109(10), 1309-34.

[33] Niddam, D. M., Tsai, S. Y., Lu, C. L., Ko, C. W., Hsieh, J. C. (2011). Reduced hippocampal glutamate-glutamine levels in irritable bowel syndrome: preliminary findings using magnetic resonance spectroscopy. *Am. J. Gastroenterol.*, 106(8), 1503-11.

[34] Apkarian, A. V., Bushnell, M. C., Treede, R. D., Zubieta, J. K. (2005). Human brain mechanisms of pain perception and regulation in health and disease. *Eur. J. Pain*, 9(4), 463-84.

[35] Derbyshire, S. W. (2003). A systematic review of neuroimaging data during visceral stimulation. *Am. J. Gastroenterol.*, 98(1), 12-20.

[36] Kupers, R., Kehlet, H. (2006). Brain imaging of clinical pain states: a critical review and strategies for future studies. *Lancet Neurol.*, 5(12), 1033-44.

[37] Tracey, I., Mantyh, P. W. (2007). The cerebral signature for pain perception and its modulation. *Neuron*, 55(3), 377-91.

[38] May, A. (2008). Chronic pain may change the structure of the brain. *Pain*, 137(1), 7-15.

[39] Gureje, O., Von Korff, M., Kola, L., Demyttenaere, K., He, Y., Posada-Villa, J., et al. (2008). The relation between multiple pains and mental disorders: results from the World Mental Health Surveys. *Pain*, 135(1-2), 82-91.

[40] Ingvar, M. (1999). Pain and functional imaging. *Philos. Trans. R Soc. Lond. B Biol. Sci.*, 354(1387), 1347-58.

[41] Heavner, J. E. (1999). Newer Concepts in Pain Mechanisms. *Curr. Rev. Pain*, 3(6), 453-7.

[42] Peyron, R., Laurent, B., Garcia-Larrea, L. (2000). Functional imaging of brain responses to pain. A review and meta-analysis (2000). *Neurophysiol. Clin.*, 30(5), 263-88.

[43] Albe-Fessard, D., Berkley, K. J., Kruger, L., Ralston, H. J., 3rd, Willis, W. D., Jr. (1985). Diencephalic mechanisms of pain sensation. *Brain Res.*, 356(3), 217-96.

[44] Mazzola, L., Isnard, J., Mauguiere, F. (2006). Somatosensory and pain responses to stimulation of the second somatosensory area (SII) in humans. A comparison with SI and insular responses. *Cereb. Cortex*, 16 (7), 960-8.

[45] Vogt, B. A., Berger, G. R., Derbyshire, S. W. (2003). Structural and functional dichotomy of human midcingulate cortex. *Eur. J. Neurosci.*, 18(11), 3134-44.

[46] Craig, A. D. (2003). Interoception: the sense of the physiological condition of the body. *Curr. Opin. Neurobiol.*, 13(4), 500-5.

[47] Niddam, D. M., Hsieh, J. C. (2009). Neuroimaging of muscle pain in humans. *J. Chin. Med. Assoc.*, 72(6), 285-93.

[48] Lu, C. L., Wu, Y. T., Yeh, T. C., Chen, L. F., Chang, F. Y., Lee, S. D., et al. (2004). Neuronal correlates of gastric pain induced by fundus distension: a 3T-fMRI study. *Neurogastroenterol. Motil.*, 16(5), 575-87.

[49] Saper, C. B. (2002). The central autonomic nervous system: conscious visceral perception and autonomic pattern generation. *Annu. Rev. Neurosci.*, 25, 433-69.

[50] Craig, A. D. (2002). How do you feel? Interoception: the sense of the physiological condition of the body. *Nat. Rev. Neurosci.*, 3(8), 655-66.

[51] Willis, W. D., Al-Chaer, E. D., Quast, M. J., Westlund, K. N. (1999). A visceral pain pathway in the dorsal column of the spinal cord. *Proc. Natl. Acad. Sci. US,* 96(14), 7675-9.

[52] Lu, H. C., Hsieh, J. C., Lu, C. L., Niddam, D. M., Wu, Y. T., Yeh, T. C., et al. (2010). Neuronal correlates in the modulation of placebo analgesia in experimentally-induced esophageal pain: a 3T-fMRI study. *Pain*, 148(1), 75-83.

[53] Mayer, E. A., Berman, S., Suyenobu, B., Labus, J., Mandelkern, M. A., Naliboff, B. D., et al. (2005). Differences in brain responses to visceral pain between patients with irritable bowel syndrome and ulcerative colitis. *Pain*, 115(3), 398-409.

[54] Silverman, D. H., Munakata, J. A., Ennes, H., Mandelkern, M. A., Hoh, C. K., Mayer, E. A. (1997). Regional cerebral activity in normal and

pathological perception of visceral pain. *Gastroenterology*, 112(1), 64-72.

[55] Verne, G. N., Himes, N. C., Robinson, M. E., Gopinath, K. S., Briggs, R. W., Crosson, B., et al. (2003). Central representation of visceral and cutaneous hypersensitivity in the irritable bowel syndrome. *Pain*, 103(1-2), 99-110.

[56] Mertz, H., Morgan, V., Tanner, G., Pickens, D., Price, R., Shyr, Y., et al. (2000). Regional cerebral activation in irritable bowel syndrome and control subjects with painful and nonpainful rectal distention. *Gastroenterology*, 118(5), 842-8.

[57] Hobson, A. R., Furlong, P. L., Worthen, S. F., Hillebrand, A., Barnes, G. R., Singh, K. D., et al. (2005). Real-time imaging of human cortical activity evoked by painful esophageal stimulation. *Gastroenterology*, 128(3), 610-9.

[58] Strigo, I. A., Duncan, G. H., Boivin, M., Bushnell, M. C. (2003). Differentiation of visceral and cutaneous pain in the human brain. *J. Neurophysiol.*, 89(6), 3294-303.

[59] Kern, M. K., Birn, R. M., Jaradeh, S., Jesmanowicz, A., Cox, R. W., Hyde, J. S., et al. (1998). Identification and characterization of cerebral cortical response to esophageal mucosal acid exposure and distention. *Gastroenterology*, 115(6), 1353-62.

[60] Aziz, Q., Andersson, J. L., Valind, S., Sundin, A., Hamdy, S., Jones, A. K., et al. (1997). Identification of human brain loci processing esophageal sensation using positron emission tomography. *Gastroenterology*, 113(1), 50-9.

[61] Van Oudenhove, L., Vandenberghe, J., Dupont, P., Geeraerts, B., Vos, R., Dirix, S., et al. (2010). Abnormal regional brain activity during rest and (anticipated) gastric distension in functional dyspepsia and the role of anxiety: a H(2)(15)O-PET study. *Am. J. Gastroenterol.*, 105(4), 913-24.

[62] Vandenberghe, J., Dupont, P., Van Oudenhove, L., Bormans, G., Demyttenaere, K., Fischler, B., et al. (2007). Regional cerebral blood flow during gastric balloon distention in functional dyspepsia. *Gastroenterology*, 132(5), 1684-93.

[63] Vandenbergh, J., Dupont, P., Fischler, B., Bormans, G., Persoons, P., Janssens, J., et al. (2005). Regional brain activation during proximal stomach distention in humans: A positron emission tomography study. *Gastroenterology*, 128(3), 564-73.

[64] Ladabaum, U., Minoshima, S., Hasler, W. L., Cross, D., Chey, W. D., Owyang, C. (2001). Gastric distention correlates with activation of multiple cortical and subcortical regions. *Gastroenterology*, 120(2), 369-76.

[65] Valfre, W., Rainero, I., Bergui, M., Pinessi, L. (2008). Voxel-based morphometry reveals gray matter abnormalities in migraine. *Headache*, 48(1), 109-17.

[66] Schmidt-Wilcke, T., Ganssbauer, S., Neuner, T., Bogdahn, U., May, A. (2008). Subtle grey matter changes between migraine patients and healthy controls. *Cephalalgia*, 28 (1), 1-4.

[67] Schmidt-Wilcke, T., Leinisch, E., Straube, A., Kampfe, N., Draganski, B., Diener, H. C., et al. (2005). Gray matter decrease in patients with chronic tension type headache. *Neurology*, 65(9), 1483-6.

[68] Schmidt-Wilcke, T., Leinisch, E., Ganssbauer, S., Draganski, B., Bogdahn, U., Altmeppen, J., et al. (2006). Affective components and intensity of pain correlate with structural differences in gray matter in chronic back pain patients. *Pain*, 125(1-2), 89-97.

[69] Apkarian, A. V., Sosa, Y., Sonty, S., Levy, R. M., Harden, R. N., Parrish, T. B., et al. (2004). Chronic back pain is associated with decreased prefrontal and thalamic gray matter density. *J. Neurosci.*, 24 (46), 10410-5.

[70] Blankstein, U., Chen, J., Diamant, N. E., Davis, K. D. (2010). Altered brain structure in irritable bowel syndrome: potential contributions of pre-existing and disease-driven factors. *Gastroenterology*, 138(5), 1783-9.

[71] Davis, K. D., Pope, G., Chen, J., Kwan, C. L., Crawley, A. P., Diamant, N. E. (2008). Cortical thinning in IBS: implications for homeostatic, attention, and pain processing. *Neurology*, 70(2), 153-4.

[72] Schweinhardt, P., Kuchinad, A., Pukall, C. F., Bushnell, M. C. (2008). Increased gray matter density in young women with chronic vulvar pain. *Pain*, 140(3), 411-9.

[73] Teutsch, S., Herken, W., Bingel, U., Schoell, E., May, A. (2008). Changes in brain gray matter due to repetitive painful stimulation. *Neuroimage*, 42(2), 845-9.

[74] Lutz, J., Jager, L., de Quervain, D., Krauseneck, T., Padberg, F., Wichnalek, M., et al. (2008). White and gray matter abnormalities in the brain of patients with fibromyalgia: a diffusion-tensor and volumetric imaging study. *Arthritis Rheum.*, 58(12), 3960-9.

[75] Gustin, S. M., Wrigley, P. J., Siddall, P. J., Henderson, L. A. (2010). Brain anatomy changes associated with persistent neuropathic pain following spinal cord injury. *Cereb. Cortex*, 20(6), 1409-19.

[76] Chen, J. Y., Blankstein, U., Diamant, N. E., Davis, K. D. (2011). White matter abnormalities in irritable bowel syndrome and relation to individual factors. *Brain Res.*, 1392, 121-31.

[77] Susumu, M., Setsu, W., Nagae-Poetscher, M. L., van Ziji, P. C. M. *MRI Atlas of Human White Matter*. 1st ed. Amsterdam, The Netherlands: Elsevier; 2005. 239 p.

[78] Lemon, R. N., Griffiths, J. (2005). Comparing the function of the corticospinal system in different species: organizational differences for motor specialization? *Muscle Nerve*, 32(3), 261-79.

[79] Wakana, S., Jiang, H., Nagae-Poetscher, L. M., van Zijl, P. C., Mori, S. (2004). Fiber tract-based atlas of human white matter anatomy. *Radiology*, 230(1), 77-87.

[80] Jones, E. G. *The Thalamus*. 2nd ed. Cambriage: Cmabriage University Press; 2007. 1644 p.

[81] Shimo, K., Ueno, T., Younger, J., Nishihara, M., Inoue, S., Ikemoto, T., et al. (2011). Visualization of painful experiences believed to trigger the activation of affective and emotional brain regions in subjects with low back pain. *PLoS ONE*, 6(11), e26681.

[82] Kulkarni, B., Bentley, D. E., Elliott, R., Julyan, P. J., Boger, E., Watson, A., et al. (2007). Arthritic pain is processed in brain areas concerned with emotions and fear. *Arthritis Rheum.*, 56(4), 1345-54.

[83] Baliki, M. N., Chialvo, D. R., Geha, P. Y., Levy, R. M., Harden, R. N., Parrish, T. B., et al. (2006). Chronic pain and the emotional brain: specific brain activity associated with spontaneous fluctuations of intensity of chronic back pain. *J. Neurosci.*, 26(47), 12165-73.

[84] Lorenz, J., Minoshima, S., Casey, K. L. (2003). Keeping pain out of mind: the role of the dorsolateral prefrontal cortex in pain modulation. *Brain*, 126(5), 1079-91.

[85] Al-Chaer, E. D., Feng, Y., Willis, W. D. (1998). A role for the dorsal column in nociceptive visceral input into the thalamus of primates. *J. Neurophysiol.*, 79(6), 3143-50.

[86] Ness, T. J. (2000). Evidence for ascending visceral nociceptive information in the dorsal midline and lateral spinal cord. *Pain*, 87(1), 83-8.

[87] Jasmin, L., Burkey, A. R., Granato, A., Ohara, P. T. (2004). Rostral agranular insular cortex and pain areas of the central nervous system: a tract-tracing study in the rat. *J. Comp. Neurol.*, 468(3), 425-40.

[88] Carmichael, S. T., Price, J. L. (1995). Sensory and premotor connections of the orbital and medial prefrontal cortex of macaque monkeys. *J. Comp. Neurol.*, 363(4), 642-64.

[89] Palecek, J., Willis, W. D. (2003). The dorsal column pathway facilitates visceromotor responses to colorectal distention after colon inflammation in rats. *Pain*, 104(3), 501-7.

[90] Saab, C. Y., Park, Y. C., Al-Chaer, E. D. (2004). Thalamic modulation of visceral nociceptive processing in adult rats with neonatal colon irritation. *Brain Res.*, 1008(2), 186-92.

[91] Romanski, L. M., Giguere, M., Bates, J. F., Goldman-Rakic, P. S. (1997). Topographic organization of medial pulvinar connections with the prefrontal cortex in the rhesus monkey. *J. Comp. Neurol.*, 379(3), 313-32.

[92] O'Doherty, J., Kringelbach, M. L., Rolls, E. T., Hornak, J., Andrews, C. (2001). Abstract reward and punishment representations in the human orbitofrontal cortex. *Nat. Neurosci.*, 4(1), 95-102.

[93] Ham, E. A., Cirillo, V. J., Zanetti, M. E., Kuehl, F. A., Jr. (1975). Estrogen-directed synthesis of specific prostaglandins in uterus. *Proc. Natl. Acad. Sci. US*, 72(4), 1420-4.

[94] Ylikorkala, O., Puolakka, J., Kauppila, A. (1979). Serum gonadotrophins, prolactin and ovarian steroids in primary dysmenorrhoea. *BJOG*, 86(8), 648-53.

[95] Suzuki, R., Rygh, L. J., Dickenson, A. H. (2004). Bad news from the brain: descending 5-HT pathways that control spinal pain processing. *Trends Pharmacol. Sci.*, 25(12), 613-7.

[96] Ulrich-Lai, Y. M., Xie, W., Meij, J. T., Dolgas, C. M., Yu, L., Herman, J. P. (2006). Limbic and HPA axis function in an animal model of chronic neuropathic pain. *Physiol. Behav.*, 88(1-2), 67-76.

[97] Kringelbach, M. L., Rolls, E. T. (2004). The functional neuroanatomy of the human orbitofrontal cortex: evidence from neuroimaging and neuropsychology. *Prog. Neurobiol.*, 72(5), 341-72.

[98] Hutton, C., Draganski, B., Ashburner, J., Weiskopf, N. (2009). A comparison between voxel-based cortical thickness and voxel-based morphometry in normal aging. *Neuroimage*, 48(2), 371-80.

[99] Sowell, E. R., Thompson, P. M., Leonard, C. M., Welcome, S. E., Kan, E., Toga, A. W. (2004). Longitudinal mapping of cortical thickness and brain growth in normal children. *J. Neurosci.*, 24(38), 8223-31.

[100] Wang, L., Wang, X., Wang, W., Chen, C., Ronnennberg, A. G., Guang, W., et al. (2004). Stress and dysmenorrhoea: a population based prospective study. *Occup. Environ. Med.*, 61(12), 1021-6.

[101] Heitkemper, M., Jarrett, M., Bond, E. F., Turner, P. (1991). GI symptoms, function, and psychophysiological arousal in dysmenorrheic women. *Nurs. Res.*, 40(1), 20-6.

[102] Vincent, K., Warnaby, C., Stagg, C. J., Moore, J., Kennedy, S., Tracey, I. (2011). Dysmenorrhoea is associated with central changes in otherwise healthy women. *Pain*, 152(9), 1966-75.

[103] McEwen, B. S. (2007). Physiology and neurobiology of stress and adaptation: central role of the brain. *Physiol. Rev.*, 87(3), 873-904.

[104] Hollis, F., Isgor, C., Kabbaj, M. (2012). The consequences of adolescent chronic unpredictable stress exposure on brain and behavior. *Neuroscience*, doi: 10.1016/j.neuroscience.2012.09.018.

[105] Archer, T. (2011). Effects of exogenous agents on brain development: stress, abuse and therapeutic compounds. *CNS Neurosci. Ther.*, 17(5), 470-89.

[106] Karlsson, L., Karlsson, H. (2010). Trauma and the adolescent brain. *Nord. J. Psychiatry*, 64(1), 3.

[107] Eiland, L., Romeo, R. D. (2012). Stress and the developing adolescent brain. *Neuroscience*, doi: 10.1016/j.neuroscience.2012.10.048.

[108] Leussis, M. P., Andersen, S. L. (2008). Is adolescence a sensitive period for depression? Behavioral and neuroanatomical findings from a social stress model. *Synapse*, 62(1), 22-30.

[109] Radley, J. J., Rocher, A. B., Janssen, W. G., Hof, P. R., McEwen, B. S., Morrison, J. H. (2005). Reversibility of apical dendritic retraction in the rat medial prefrontal cortex following repeated stress. *Exp. Neurol.*, 196 (1), 199-203.

[110] Radley, J. J., Morrison, J. H. (2005). Repeated stress and structural plasticity in the brain. *Ageing Res. Rev.*, 4(2), 271-87.

[111] As-Sanie, S., Harris, R. E., Napadow, V., Kim, J., Neshewat, G., Kairys, A., et al. (2012). Changes in regional gray matter volume in women with chronic pelvic pain: a voxel-based morphometry study. *Pain*, 153(5), 1006-14.

[112] Adewuya, A. O., Loto, O. M., Adewumi, T. A. (2008). Premenstrual dysphoric disorder amongst Nigerian university students: prevalence,

comorbid conditions, and correlates. *Archives Women's Ment Health*, 11 (1), 13-8.

[113] Blanchard, E. B., Lackner, J. M., Jaccard, J., Rowell, D., Carosella, A. M., Powell, C., et al. (2008). The role of stress in symptom exacerbation among IBS patients. *J. Psychosom. Res.*, 64(2), 119-28.

[114] Chang, L., Sundaresh, S., Elliott, J., Anton, P. A., Baldi, P., Licudine, A., et al. (2009). Dysregulation of the hypothalamic-pituitary-adrenal (HPA) axis in irritable bowel syndrome. *Neurogastroenterol. Motil.*, 21 (2), 149-59.

[115] Grandi, G., Ferrari, S., Xholli, A., Cannoletta, M., Palma, F., Romani, C., et al. (2012). Prevalence of menstrual pain in young women: what is dysmenorrhea? *J. Pain Res.*, 5, 169-74.

[116] Gumanga, S. K., Kwame-Aryee, R. A. (2012). Menstrual characteristics in some adolescent girls in Accra, Ghana. *Ghana Med. J.*, 46(1), 3-7.

[117] Karout, N., Hawai, S. M., Altuwaijri, S. (2012). Prevalence and pattern of menstrual disorders among Lebanese nursing students. *East Mediterr. Health J.*, 18(4), 346-52.

[118] Santina, T., Wehbe, N., Ziade, F. (2012). Exploring dysmenorrhoea and menstrual experiences among Lebanese female adolescents. *East Mediterr. Health J.*, 18(8), 857-63.

[119] Muhammad, Y. Y., Nossier, S. A., El-Dawaiaty, A. A. (2011). Prevalence and characteristics of chronic pelvic pain among women in Alexandria, Egypt. *J. Egypt Public Health Assoc.*, 86(1-2), 33-8.

[120] Omidvar, S., Begum, K. (2011). Menstrual pattern among unmarried women from south India. *J. Nat. Sci. Biol. Med.*, 2(2), 174-9.

[121] Tavallaee, M., Joffres, M. R., Corber, S. J., Bayanzadeh, M., Rad, M. M. (2011). The prevalence of menstrual pain and associated risk factors among Iranian women. *J. Obstet. Gynaecol. Res.*, 37(5), 442-51.

[122] Wong, L. P. (2011). Attitudes towards dysmenorrhoea, impact and treatment seeking among adolescent girls: a rural school-based survey. *Aust. J. Rural Health*, 19(4), 218-23.

[123] Agarwal, A. K., Agarwal, A. (2010). A study of dysmenorrhea during menstruation in adolescent girls. *Indian J. Community Med.*, 35(1), 159-64.

[124] Al-Kindi, R., Al-Bulushi, A. (2011). Prevalence and Impact of Dysmenorrhoea among Omani High School Students. Sultan Qaboos *Univ. Med. J.*, 11(4), 485-91.

[125] Eryilmaz, G., Ozdemir, F., Pasinlioglu, T. (2010). Dysmenorrhea prevalence among adolescents in eastern Turkey: its effects on school

performance and relationships with family and friends. *J. Pediatr. Adolesc. Gynecol.*, 23(5), 267-72.

[126] Ortiz, M. I. (2010). Primary dysmenorrhea among Mexican university students: prevalence, impact and treatment. *Eur. J. Obstet. Gynecol. Reprod. Biol.*, 152(1), 73-7.

[127] Parker, M. A., Sneddon, A. E., Arbon, P. (2010). The menstrual disorder of teenagers (MDOT) study: determining typical menstrual patterns and menstrual disturbance in a large population-based study of Australian teenagers. *BJOG*, 117(2), 185-92.

[128] Unsal, A., Ayranci, U., Tozun, M., Arslan, G., Calik, E. (2010). Prevalence of dysmenorrhea and its effect on quality of life among a group of female university students. *Ups. J. Med. Sci.*, 115(2), 138-45.

[129] Chan, S. C., Yiu, K. W., Yuen, P. M., Sahota, D. S., Chung, K. H. (2009). Menstrual problems and health-seeking behaviour in Hong Kong Chinese girls. *Hong Kong Med. J.*, 15(1), 18-23.

[130] Fawole, A. O., Babarinsa, I. A., Fawole, O. I., Obisesan, K. A., Ojengbede, O. A. (2009). Menstrual characteristics of secondary school girls in Ibadan, Nigeria. *West Afr. J. Med.*, 28(2), 92-6.

[131] Yamamoto, K., Okazaki, A., Sakamoto, Y., Funatsu, M. (2009). The relationship between premenstrual symptoms, menstrual pain, irregular menstrual cycles, and psychosocial stress among Japanese college students. *J. Physiol. Anthropol.*, 28(3), 129-36.

[132] Zegeye, D. T., Megabiaw, B., Mulu, A. (2009). Age at menarche and the menstrual pattern of secondary school adolescents in northwest Ethiopia. *BMC Women's Health*, 9, 29.

[133] Pitts, M. K., Ferris, J. A., Smith, A. M., Shelley, J. M., Richters, J. (2008). Prevalence and correlates of three types of pelvic pain in a nationally representative sample of Australian women. *Med. J. Aust.*, 189(3), 138-43.

[134] Sharma, P., Malhotra, C., Taneja, D. K., Saha, R. (2008). Problems related to menstruation amongst adolescent girls. *Indian J. Pediatr.*, 75 (2), 125-9.

[135] Ortiz, M. I., Fernandez-Martinez, E., Perez-Hernandez, N., Macias, A., Rangel-Flores, E., Ponce-Monter, H. (2007). Patterns of prescription and self-medication for treating primary dysmenorrhea in a Mexican population. *Proc. West Pharmacol. Soc.*, 50, 165-7.

[136] Gurel, H., Atar Gurel, S. (1999). Dyspareunia, back pain and chronic pelvic pain: the importance of this pain complex in gynecological

practice and its relation with grandmultiparity and pelvic relaxation. *Gynecol. Obstet. Invest.*, 48(2), 119-22.

[137] Harlow, S. D., Park, M. (1996). A longitudinal study of risk factors for the occurrence, duration and severity of menstrual cramps in a cohort of college women. *BJOG*, 103(11), 1134-42.

[138] Jamieson, D. J., Steege, J. F. (1996). The prevalence of dysmenorrhea, dyspareunia, pelvic pain, and irritable bowel syndrome in primary care practices. *Obstet. Gynecol.*, 87(1), 55-8.

[139] Ng, T. P., Tan, N. C., Wansaicheong, G. K. (1992). A prevalence study of dysmenorrhoea in female residents aged 15-54 years in Clementi Town, Singapore. *Ann. Acad. Med. Singapore*, 21(3), 323-7.

[140] Sundell, G., Milsom, I., Andersch, B. (1990). Factors influencing the prevalence and severity of dysmenorrhoea in young women. *BJOG*, 97 (7), 588-94.

[141] Thomas, K. D., Okonofua, F. E., Chiboka, O. (1990). A study of the menstrual patterns of adolescents in Ile-Ife, Nigeria. *Int. J. Gynaecol. Obstet.*, 33(1), 31-4.

[142] Pullon, S., Reinken, J., Sparrow, M. (1988). Prevalence of dysmenorrhoea in Wellington women. *N Z Med. J.*, 101(839), 52-4.

[143] Andersch, B., Milsom, I. (1982). An epidemiologic study of young women with dysmenorrhea. *Am. J. Obstet. Gynecol.*, 144(6), 655-60.

In: Menstrual Cycle
Editor: Madeleine Gosselin

ISBN: 978-1-62417-945-7
© 2013 Nova Science Publishers, Inc.

Chapter III

Toward a More Comprehensive View of Premenstrual Disorders: The Case for Psychological Contributions

***Julia R. Craner and Sandra T. Sigmon**[*]*
University of Maine, Orono, ME, US

Abstract

Premenstrual disorders include premenstrual dysphoric disorder (PMDD) and premenstrual syndrome (PMS). Unlike commonly occurring premenstrual symptoms, premenstrual disorders involve severe affective, behavioral, and physiological symptoms that cause distress and impairment. Research on purely biological causes for premenstrual diosrders has been unequivocal to date. Consequently, a promising area of research is to explore the role of psychological factors that may interact with physiological changes and contribute to the development and maintenance of PMS and PMDD. The current chapter focuses on psychological contributions to premenstrual distress, which are supported

[*] Corresponding author: Sandra Sigmon, PhD. 301 Little Hall. Department of Psychology, University of Maine, Orono, ME 04469. Ph: 207-581-2049. Fax: 207-581-6128. E-mail: Sandra.sigmon@umit.maine.edu.

by the following: 1) symptom overlap and comorbidity between premenstrual disorders and psychological disorders, 2) premenstrual exacerbation of underlying psychological conditions, 3) the potential role of self-focused attention and coping in premenstrual disorders, and 4) symptom improvement as a result of psychological interventions. A holistic approach to premenstrual symptoms and disorders, involving biological, psychological, and social factors, provides a more comprehensive understanding of these disorders that has important implications for research and treatment.

Premenstrual distress typically involves affective, behavioral, and physical symptoms. In women with premenstrual disorders, including premenstrual syndrome (PMS) and premenstrual dysphoric disorder (PMDD), these symptoms are severe enough to cause distress and interfere in daily functioning. The majority of research on premenstrual symptoms and disorders has focused on biological factors, such as endocrine functioning. However, results have been mixed and inconsistent, suggesting that biological explanations alone are not sufficient. Although the menstrual cycle is associated with physiological changes, psychological factors may interact with these changes in a manner that increases distress, particularly in women with premenstrual disorders. This is a promising area of research that is consistent with biopsychosocial approaches to health and wellbeing. Evidence supporting the role of psychological contributions in premenstrual disorders is drawn from the significant symptom overlap and comorbidity between premenstrual and psychological concerns, premenstrual exacerbation of symptoms in other disorders, the potential role of self-focused attention and coping in premenstrual disorders, and improvement in symptoms as a result of psychological interventions.

Premenstrual Symptoms and Disorders

The menstrual cycle is a natural physiological process, and menstrual cycle-related changes are commonly reported in the general population. Approximately 80% of women report noticing premenstrual symptoms (Sigmon, Craner, Yoon, & Thorpe, 2012). However, for some women, premenstrual symptoms are severe enough that they cause distress and impairment. These symptoms may include premenstrual exacerbation of underlying conditions (e.g., anxiety disorders, depression, health conditions) as well as core premenstrual disorders (O'Brien et al., 2011). Core premenstrual disorders include premenstrual syndrome (PMS) and premenstrual dysphoric disorder (PMDD; O'Brien et al., 2011). These disorders are characterized by a specific cyclical pattern of symptoms; symptoms arise during the premenstrual phase, remit within a few days of the onset of menstruation, and are not present during the remainder of the menstrual cycle (APA, 2000; Sigmon et al., 2012). In addition, premenstrual disorders remit after menopause, during pregnancy, or during other interruptions of the ovulatory cycle (Di Guilio & Reissing, 2006). Although symptoms of other conditions may be exacerbated premenstrually or occur comorbidly, PMS and PMDD criteria require that these disorders do not simply represent an exacerbation of another condition (O'Brien et al., 2011). The unique cyclical pattern in premenstrual disorders differentiates them from other disorders.

Symptoms of premenstrual disorders include physical (e.g., bloating, breast tenderness, headache), behavioral (e.g., social withdrawal), and affective symptoms (e.g., mood swings, irritability; Yonkers, O'Brien, & Eriksson, 2008). Although PMS and PMDD share typical symptoms, PMDD is differentiated by more severe symptoms, including prominent affective symptoms (e.g., Clayton, 2008). Although not an exhaustive list, the most common premenstrual symptoms reported in premenstrual disorders include: physical symptoms, food cravings, low sex drive, mood swings, appetite changes, sadness/tearfulness, irritability, sensitivity to rejection, being easily upset, performance difficulties at work, feeling "on edge," depressed mood, relationship problems, social isolation, and concentration difficulties (Hartlage et al., 2012).

The term PMS is widely used to describe women with premenstrual changes (Markens, 1996), but more precisely, PMS represents a clinically significant category of premenstrual distress. Women with PMS report experiencing at least one moderate to severe symptom occurring during the premenstrual phase (Andrzej & Diana, 2006). There is no universally agreed upon number or severity of symptoms, and prevalence estimates vary widely based on different criteria and assessment methods (e.g., Sigmon et al., 2012). Although some researchers suggest that when rigorous criteria are applied using prospective assessment, 5-8% of women can be categorized as having PMS, other researchers have suggested that closer to 20-40% of women experience clinically significant premenstrual symptoms qualifying for PMS diagnosis (Halbreich, Borenstein, Pearlstein, & Kahn, 2003; O'Brien et al., 2011; Yonkers et al., 2008). PMDD is less prevalent than PMS, and is estimated to affect 2-5% of premenopausal women (Epperson et al., 2012).

This disorder is characterized by marked depressed mood, anxiety, mood changes, and decreased interest in usual activities that are severe enough to impair functioning and cause distress (Yonkers et al., 2003). Diagnostic criteria for PMDD require at least five moderate to severe symptoms, with at least one of those symptoms being a severe affective symptom (i.e., depressed mood, loss of interest, anger/irritability, anxiety, or mood swings). Although PMDD is currently diagnosed as a mood disorder, research indicates that anger/irritability, anxiety/tension, fatigue/lethargy, and mood swings are reported more often than sadness/depression in women with PMDD (e.g., Pearlstein, Yonkers, Fayyad, & Gillespie, 2005). The International Society for Premenstrual Disorders (ISPMD) formed a consensus group to initiate a unified diagnostic approach to premenstrual distress. These disorders were broadly lumped together as "premenstrual disorders," or PMD. PMD includes PMS, PMDD, as well as significant premenstrual symptoms that do not qualify for other disorders (O'Brien et al., 2011). An advantage of this broad label is that it allows for a discussion of premenstrual distress in general, and avoids the pitfalls of rigidly applying diagnostic labels that are often controversial and poorly defined.

Premenstrual disorders are present in adolescents and premenopausal adult women. There is mixed evidence concerning age of onset. Research suggests that severe symptoms most typically emerge around age 26 (Davis & Yonkers, 1997); however, other studies have not found a significant relationship between age and PMDD diagnosis (Tschudin, Bertea, & Zemp, 2010) or have found similar prevalence rates in adolescent samples as in adult samples (Steiner et al., 2011). Typically women with premenstrual disorders experience a similar symptom pattern during each premenstrual phase (Yonkers et al., 2008) that follows a chronic course (Wittchen, Becker, Lieb, & Krause, 2002). This suggests that a considerable proportion of menstruating women across age groups are impacted by premenstrual distress.

In women with premenstrual disorders, premenstrual symptoms are associated with significant impairment in numerous areas of functioning. Research indicates that women high in premenstrual distress report dissatisfaction with social relationships, impaired social adjustment, and increased interpersonal difficulties during the premenstrual phase (Di Guilio & Reissing, 2006). Nevertheless, there is some evidence that women with PMDD experience more social impairment than controls, including during the follicular phase, despite being relatively asymptomatic during that phase (Pearlstein et al., 2000). Most notably, in women with PMDD, 15% report at least one suicide attempt (Cunningham, Yonkers, O'Brien, & Eriksson, 2009).

Other researchers have found increased impairment in home, social, and family functioning compared to work functioning (Halbreich et al., 2003; Robinson & Swindle, 2000). However, premenstrual symptoms may also interfere with occupational functioning. Researchers found that women with PMDD reported decreased productivity during the premenstrual phase compared to women with minimal symptoms (Chawla, Swindle, Long, Kennedy & Sterfield, 2002). Additionally, researchers have found that moderate to severe premenstrual symptoms are associated with reduced occupational productivity and more frequent absenteeism at work (Borenstein, Dean, Leifke, Kornet, Yonkers, 2007). Cognitive impairments are often reported in women with PMS and PMDD (e.g., Cortina, 2005). Women with high premenstrual distress tend to report a subjective sense of increased difficulty with attention, memory, and motor coordination during the premenstrual phase (Cortina, 2005). However, in studies investigating PMS/PMDD and cognitive performance, results have been mixed. Overall, there do not appear to be any significant differences in learning, attention, or memory in premenstrual women, regardless of whether or not they experience PMS/PMDD (Cortina, 2005; Resnick, Perry, Parry, Mostofi, & Udell, 1998). Thus, reports of cognitive impairments could be related to the perception of symptoms and/or the attribution of cognitive symptoms to the menstrual cycle, although more research is needed.

Research on health-related quality of life has found that both PMS and PMDD are related to a significant health-related quality of life burden (Borenstein et al., 2007; Yang et al., 2008). In one study comparing health-related quality of life scores for women with abnormal and painful menstrual cycles and severe premenstrual symptoms, all three groups reported lower physical health status than the women without menstrual symptoms; however, the women with premenstrual symptoms reported the lowest mental health-related quality of life compared to the other groups (Barnard, Frayne, Skinner, & Sullivan, 2003). Other researchers have suggested that the overall health burden of PMDD is comparable to other chronic conditions, such as arthritis (Yang et al., 2008). Although women with premenstrual disorders report greater overall health care utilization than controls (Borenstein et al., 2007), research indicates that women with PMS or PMDD likely have unmet medical needs for their premenstrual symptoms. This finding may be due to lack of treatment-seeking behavior for premenstrual symptoms (Hylan, Sundell, & Judge, 1999), which may also be influenced by personal and societal perceptions of premenstrual disorders, including lack of awareness of its associated impairment. For example, the World Health Organization (WHO,

2001) report on the significant health burden of mental health issues did not include categories of PMS or PMDD. Given that the current classification system of psychological disorders (i.e., DSM-IV-TR; APA, 2000) places PMDD in the appendix (rather than a formal diagnostic category), and does not list PMS, this may also contribute to lack of recognition for the validity of PMDD as a disorder (Pearlstein, 2010). This may change in the future as classification systems are updated.

Overall, PMS and PMDD represent cyclical disorders in women that are associated with distress and impact functioning. These premenstrual disorders represent disturbances menstrual cycle-related symptoms, and affect a significant proportion of women. Accordingly, premenstrual disorders and symptoms are an important area for study. Perhaps in part because research on women's health issues have lagged behind that of men, little is known about the underlying causes of PMS and PMDD.

Etiological Theories and Research

Premenstrual disorders involve significant physical, psychological, and behavioral changes that occur cyclically during the premenstrual phase, and remit for the remainder of the menstrual cycle. This cyclical pattern of changes continues to perplex researchers, and many models have been proposed to account for these disorders. These explanations include biological social, and psychological theories of etiology; however, no one theory has been successful in accounting for these disorders based on the current state of research in the field.

It is clear that the onset of symptoms in PMS and PMDD correspond with physiological menstrual cycle changes. During the premenstrual phase of the menstrual cycle, there is a dramatic decrease in levels of ovarian steroid hormones, including both estrogen and progesterone (e.g., Cunningham et al., 2009). Thus, the majority of research has focused on biological explanations for premenstrual disorders. Researchers have hypothesized that women with premenstrual disorders have differences in gonadal hormone levels or endocrine functioning. This view is supported by evidence that symptoms are not typically present during interruptions of the ovulatory cycle (e.g., pregnancy, ovariectomy), and other some studies have found that hormonal contraceptive may be an effective treatment for premenstrual symptoms (e.g., Di Guilio & Reissing, 2006). However, research findings have been mixed, and no clear or convincing evidence has been presented that suggests that there are any hormonal differences in women with and without premenstrual disorders (Davis & Yonkers, 1997; Cunningham et al., 2009; Biggs & Demuth, 2011).

The contributions of neurotransmitter levels and function have also been investigated in premenstrual disorders, particularly due to the association with various neurotransmitters (e.g., serotonin, GABA) with mood and anxiety symptoms. In addition, selective serotonin reuptake inhibitors (SSRIs) have been an effective treatment for some women with premenstrual mood symptoms (Cunningham et al., 2009). However, in general, research on the role of neurotransmitters in premenstrual disorders has been mixed, and this relationship is unclear (Davis & Yonkers, 1997; Cunningham et al., 2009; Di Guilio & Reissing, 2006). This is similar to research on other affective disorders – the role of brain circuitry, including neurotransmitter function, is likely to be more complex than single neurotransmitter dysfunction (Rapkin & Akopians, 2012). There also appears to be a genetic influence in premenstrual symptoms, with a high concordance rate found in monozygotic and same-gender dizygotic twins (Jahanfar, Lye, & Krishnarajah, 2011).

In summary, there is no evidence at present that points to specific biological influences that would fully account for premenstrual disorders. This does not suggest that premenstrual symptoms are not related to physiological menstrual cycle changes. Indeed, given that the majority of women report at least one premenstrual symptom, some degree of premenstrual change is attributable to normal physiological changes rather than pathology (Yonkers et al., 2003). There is also research supporting biological bases for premenstrual disorders to some extent (for a review, see Rapkin & Akopians, 2012). However, purely biological explanations based on current research do not appear to account for the severe physical, emotional, and behavioral symptoms observed in PMS and PMDD. One possibility is that women with PMS and PMDD may be more physiologically sensitive to menstrual cycle changes, and report more symptoms associated with the premenstrual phase (Biggs & Demuth, 2011).

This hypothesis is supported by research indicating that women with PMS respond with more negative affect to hormone administrations compared to women without a history of premenstrual symptoms (Schmidt, Nieman, Danaceau, Adams, & Rubinow, 1998). Therefore, biologically-based menstrual cycle-related changes (e.g., hormone fluctuation) may serve as "triggers" for premenstrual symptoms in women who are more sensitive to these changes, rather than as causal agents in themselves.

Social models of etiology suggest that societal factors contribute to the development and/or maintenance of premenstrual disorders. Theorists have suggested that the content of what girls are taught about menstruation, as well as societal views that tend to reinforce that menstruation is painful, debilitating, or something to be embarrassed about, could contribute to premenstrual distress (Sigmon, Rohan, Boulard, Dorhofer, & Whitcomb, 2000). This hypothesis is supported by research that indicates that women report premenstrual symptoms consistent with their views on menstruation in general (MacFarland, Ross, & DeCourville, 1989). For example, resesarchers found that the more women endorsed the widespread phenomenon of premenstrual symptoms, the more they reported negative symptoms during their last premenstrual phase (MacFarland et al., 1989). Cultural factors, such as race/ethnicity and acculturation status may impact reports of premenstrual disorders. One study (Pilver, Kasl, Desai, & Levy, 2011) found that a positive relationship between PMDD symptoms and acculturation status; specifically, the reports of PMDD increased as the duration of residence in the United States increased. However, researchers have also suggested that premenstrual disorders are prevalent internationally at relatively similar rates as in the United States (e.g., Halbreich et al., 2003; Adewuya, Loto, & Adewumi, 2008), though slightly lower in Japan (Takeda, Tasaka, Sakata, Murata, 2006). Overall, cultural and social factors likely influence the experience or expression of premenstrual symptoms; however, there is not a comprehensive social theory supported by research that accounts for the etiology of premenstrual disorders.

Historically, little research has investigated psychological factors that may play a role in the development and maintenance of premenstrual disorders. Unfortunately, the current state of research into psychological contributions to premenstrual disorders lacks a research-supported comprehensive theory of etiology. Psychoanalytic explanations have focused on the meaning of the symptoms, including repressed hostility toward males or grief over failure to conceive (Davis & Yonkers, 1997). More contemporary research, however, has emphasized factors such as stress, coping styles, and personality traits. For example, research indicates that women with premenstrual disorders report higher levels of trait neuroticism (Gingnell, Camsco, Oreland, Fredrikson, & Sundstöm-Promoaa, 2010), display a negative bias toward affective content during the premenstrual phase (Rubinow, Smith, Schenkel, Schmidt, & Dancer, 2007), perceive events more negatively during the premenstrual phase (Gonda et al., 2010), report more emotion-oriented coping (Mitchell & Mitchell, 1998), and perceive daily stressors as more stressful during the premenstrual phase (Fontana & Badawy, 1997). One limitation of existing psychological research on premenstrual disorders is that it often does not account for both physical and affective symptoms involved in PMS and PMDD, as well as the cyclical nature of these symptoms. For example, underlying personality characteristics do not explain why women would only be symptomatic during the premenstrual phase.

One model, the Menstrual Reactivity Hypothesis, indicates that the menstrual cycle can be viewed as a type of cyclical stressor, and certain women may report more severe and a greater number of menstrual symptoms due to accurate reports of symptoms as well as expectations, such as cultural beliefs, sex roles, and attitudes toward physical symptoms (Sigmon et al., 2000).

Importantly, this model suggests that women's *reactions* to menstrual cycle changes may be associated with distress, corresponding to the cyclical nature of symptoms. However, this model has not been directly researched in women meeting criteria for PMS and PMDD. In addition, this model focuses on the physical symptoms involved in premenstrual distress, and may not be sufficient to explain the significant mood changes in women with premenstrual disorders, particularly in PMDD.

According to a biopsychosocial perspective, multiple factors interact to influence health and functioning. This perspective is particularly applicable to premenstrual disorders. Although menstruation is a normal physical process for women, and some degree of premenstrual change is typical, psychological factors may influence the report, interpretation, and experience of symptoms. Similarly, social and cultural factors, such as societal messages about the menstrual cycle, as well as demographic factors (e.g., race/ethnicity), may influence premenstrual symptom reporting (Sigmon et al., 2012).

In consideration that research into biological theories of etiology has not produced any conclusive results, a more holistic understanding of the causes of premenstrual disorder is warranted. One possibility is that women with PMS and PMDD are more sensitive to physiological premenstrual changes and react to these changes in a manner that tends to increase distress.

This hypothesis emphasizes the possibility that psychological contributions could play an important role in the onset and maintenance of premenstrual disorders. Although biological factors certainly play an instrumental role in premenstrual symptoms, the *interaction* between physiological changes and social and psychological factors provides a more comprehensive explanation for PMS and PMDD.

The Case for Psychological Contributions to Premenstrual Disorders

PMS and PMDD are associated with cyclical emotional, physical, and behavioral symptoms. Accordingly, it follows that psychological contributions may be involved due to the nature of the symptoms. Although there is a lack of a comprehensive model of premenstrual disorders, investigating the underlying psychological contributions that may be inflectional in these disorders could greatly add to our understanding of PMS/PMDD and build upon and integrate previous research. A case for psychological contributions is presented here, based on the following: 1) comorbidity and symptom overlap between PMS/PMDD and psychological disorders, 2) premenstrual exacerbation of symptoms in other disorders, 3) existing research on underlying psychological factors, and 4) psychological interventions.

Symptom Overlap and Comorbidity

The following are common symptoms of PMS and PMDD: anger, irritability, anxiety, depressed mood, hopelessness, tearfulness, feeling overwhelmed, decreased interest in activities, mood swings, feeling rejected, and difficulty concentrating (Steiner et al.; Epperson et al., 2012). Although significant physical symptoms are typical in women with premenstrual disorders (e.g., bloating, breast tenderness), there is a preponderance of emotional symptoms reported, particularly by women with PMDD (Pearlstein et al., 2005). Behavioral change is also associated with premenstrual symptoms, such as social withdrawal and sleep disturbance (Clayton, 2008). A significant body of research has been conducted into underlying psychological factors in disorders with primarily emotional and/or behavioral symptoms (e.g., mood and anxiety disorders); however, this has not been extended to premenstrual disorders. Despite this, comorbidity and symptom overlap between PMS/PMDD and other disorders may help provide insight into psychological contributions to premenstrual disorders.

The significant comorbidity that exists between PMS/PMDD and psychological disorders presents important diagnostic and research considerations. The comorbidity between mood disorders and PMDD is especially high, with 30-70% of women with PMDD estimated to develop depression during their lifetime (Davis & Yonkers, 1997). This comorbidity rate is high even after considering that up to 30% of women will develop some form of depression during their lifetime (Yonkers et al., 2008). Researchers have suggested that PMDD may increase a woman's risk for the development of later major depression (Hartlage, Arduino, & Gehlert, 2001). Other researchers have suggested high comorbidity rates between PMS and depression. For example, one study found that 24.6% of women with severe PMS met criteria for major depression, as well as 11.3% of women with moderate PMS (Forrester-Knauss, Stutz, Weiss, & Tschudin, 2001). Considering that the current prevalence of depression in women is approximately 10% (Centers for Disease Control and Prevention [CDC], 2012), this is a notable finding. Regarding depression history, research has found that 57.6% of women with PMDD report a history of depression (Cohen et al., 2002). A history of severe premenstrual symptoms may also increase women's risk of developing perimenopausal and postnatal depression (Yonkers et al., 2008). For example, Garcia-Esteve and colleages (2008) found that PMS was an independent risk factor for the development of postpartum depression. Overall, this suggests a significant co-occurrence of premenstrual and mood disorders.

Bipolar disorder and seasonal affective disorder (SAD) are similar to premenstrual disorders in that they also involve cyclical mood changes. There is a considerable amount of comorbidity between bipolar disorder, SAD, and premenstrual disorders. In women with bipolar disorder, research suggests that 27.2% self-report a lifetime history of PMDD (Fornaro & Perugi, 2010). Another study indicated that 65.1.-70.5% of women with bipolar disorder reported premenstrual mood symptoms, whereas 33.7% of women with no diagnosis reported these symptoms (Payne et al., 2007). In women with SAD, one study found an increase in PMDD during both symptomatic and asymptomatic seasons, and an overall comorbidity rate of 38-46% (Kim et al., 2004). Therefore, there may be underlying similarities among this group of disorders.

Anxiety disorders are also highly comorbid with premenstrual disorders. Lifetime comorbidity of anxiety disorders in women with PMDD is estimated to be about 14-15% (Davis & Yonkers, 1997). In women with PMS, researchers found that 25% of women presenting for treatment of diagnosed PMS also met diagnostic criteria for anxiety disorder (GAD) and 25% were diagnosed with comorbid panic disorder (Kim et al., 2004). Other researchers found that 15% of women with PMS also met criteria for an anxiety disorder, particularly panic disorder (9%) but also met criteria for generalized anxiety disorder and obsessive-compulsive disorder (Bailey & Cohen, 1999).

Researchers have also proposed that PMDD may be a variant of panic disorder, given that women with PMDD respond to panic-inducing biological challenges (e.g., inhaling an air mixture high in carbon dioxide) with elevated levels of panic symptoms compared to controls (Vickers & McNally, 2004). In addition, women with premenstrual distress tend to score higher than controls on measures of anxiety, even when they are not in the premenstrual phase (Veeninga, de Ruiter, & Kraaimaat, 1994). Wittchen and colleagues (2003) suggested that women with a history of trauma were more likely to have an increased risk for developing PMDD. Similar results were obtained by Pilver and colleagues (2011). These findings suggest that clinicians should assess for a past history of trauma in women presenting with PMS/PMDD.

The comorbidity rates between PMS/PMDD and psychological disorders raise important etiological issues. One possibility is that premenstrual disorders share underlying etiological similarities between premenstrual and other disorders, or shared vulnerabilities for developing such disorders. Importantly, research supports the role of biological factors contributing to mood and anxiety disorders (e.g., neurotransmitters, fight-or-flight response), as well as psychological factors that interact with these vulnerabilities. Mood and anxiety disorders also involve considerable physiological symptoms (e.g., sleep disturbance, fatigue, muscle tension, physical panic symptoms). Similar to these disorders, understanding the interaction between physical and psychological causes for premenstrual disorders could contribute to biopsychosocial models of health.

Premenstrual Exacerbation

As mentioned previously, it is difficult to distinguish between symptoms of PMS/PMDD, similar symptoms associated with co-morbid disorders, and premenstrual exacerbation of other psychological disorders. Premenstrual exacerbation (i.e., premenstrual aggravation, premenstrual magnification) refers to an increase in symptom severity and possible impairment during the premenstrual phase that occurs in other psychological disorders or medical conditions that have symptoms that are clearly distinguishable from PMS/PMDD. Indeed, PMDD criteria require that the symptom experience cannot represent an exacerbation of another psychological disorder. For example, a woman may be diagnosed with MDD and her symptoms of depression may also worsen during the premenstrual phase. However, the overlap of anxiety and mood disorder symptoms and PMDD criteria often lead to complex assessment, diagnostic and treatment decisions.

In Hartlage and Gehlert's framework (2001), research should start "differentiating PMDD from premenstrual exacerbation one symptom at a time" (pg. 245). In this process, symptoms of PMDD are differentiated from symptoms of a co-morbid disorder in a prospective assessment. If symptoms of the co-morbid disorder worsen premenstrually, then those symptoms would be conceptualized as an exacerbation of the co-morbid disorder. According to the authors, not counting overlapping symptoms of PMDD would be a conservative approach. This tactic would be similar to the one typically used in diagnosis (e.g., not diagnosing someone with two depressive disorders) and would potentially work well with disorders that do not share overlapping symptoms with PMDD (e.g., premenstrual exacerbation of binge eating). In addition, the cyclical nature of symptoms and functional impairment becomes critical in detecting the presence of premenstrual exacerbation.

Researchers have found many indications of premenstrual exacerbation in both psychological and physical conditions. Women diagnosed with panic disorder may report increases in anxious mood and more panic attacks occurring during the premenstrual phase of the menstrual cycle (Kaspi, Otto, Pollack, & Eppinger, 1994). Researchers have also found that women seeking treatment for PMS/PMDD may be more likely to be diagnosed instead with major depression or dysthymia (McMillan & Pihl, 1987). Women with other psychological disorders may also present with premenstrual exacerbation. For example, women diagnosed with schizophrenia may report increases in psychotic symptoms during the premenstrual phase (Seeman, 2012). Researchers have also found that women report increases in symptoms of generalized anxiety disorder (that do not overlap with PMS/PMDD) during the premenstrual phase (Hsiao, Hsiao, & Liu, 2004). Hourani, Yuan, and Bray (2004) found that military women reporting premenstrual symptoms were also more likely to report increased alcohol intake, migraines and health-care visits. Gladis and Walsh (1997) found that women with bulimia engaged in more binge eating during the premenstrual phase. Similarly, in a sample of non-clinical women, researchers found that women engaged in more binge eating during the premenstrual phase (Klump. Keel, Culbert, & Edler, 2008).

In addition, researchers have found premenstrual exacerbation of physical diseases and/or conditions. Research indicates that women may report more asthma attacks (Dorhofer & Sigmon, 2002), migraine headaches (Allais et al., 2012), epileptic seizures (Herzog et al., 2011), increases in Parkinson's disease symptoms (Martignoni et al., 2003) and seasonal depression symptoms

(Portella, Haaga, & Rohan, 2006) during the premenstrual phase. Clearly, more research is needed to distinguish between premenstrual exacerbation of other psychological and physical disorders and core premenstrual disorders.

Findings supporting the premenstrual exacerbation of psychological disorders, in conjunction with research on the comorbidity between these groups of disorders, support the hypothesis that the etiology of PMS/PMDD may be impacted by psychological contributions. Specifically, women with psychological disorders may be particularly susceptible to premenstrual hormonal changes that trigger symptoms. This process suggests that there are likely to be similarities between women with PMS/PMDD and other disorders that would account for this process.

Self-Focused Attention and Coping in Women with Premenstrual Symptoms

A substantial body of research indicates that the manner in which individuals cope with and respond to symptoms has implications for the outcome of those symptoms. The construct of self-focused attention has been linked to both psychological and physical symptoms and a range of clinical disorders. Self-focused attention is defined as "awareness of self-referent, internally generated information that stands in contrast to an awareness of externally generated information" (Ingram, 1990, p. 156). A range of coping strategies can be conceptualized as forms of self-focused attention (e.g., body vigilance, rumination, health anxiety, emotion-focused coping), and research has demonstrated a strong relationship between forms of self-focused attention and negative mood, anxiety, and depression (e.g., Mor & Winquist, 2002). The concept of self-focused attention may be particularly relevant for a better understanding of the experience of premenstrual disorders. The premenstrual phase of the menstrual cycle is associated with physiological and emotional fluctuations for many women; however, only certain women experience significant distress associated with premenstrual symptoms. Self-focused attention on premenstrual mood and physical changes could help account for this relationship.

Two forms of self-focused attention, anxiety sensitivity and rumination, are potential constructs that may be implicated in the etiology and maintenance of premenstrual disorders. Anxiety sensitivity is defined as fear of physical anxiety sensations (e.g., Esteve & Camacho, 2008); such as increased heart rate, dizziness, and other somatic symptoms and their consequences. Anxiety sensitivity has been linked to a variety of disorders, including panic and other anxiety disorders, depression, substance abuse, chronic pain, and maladaptive health-related behaviors (Esteve & Camacho, 2008). Anxiety sensitivity is particularly relevant to the experience of premenstrual symptoms, as increased self-focused attention to internal changes as well as negative beliefs about these symptoms may be instrumental in determining the extent to which women are affected by the menstrual cycle. This relationship could also aid in understanding high comorbidity rates between premenstrual disorders and other disorders, particularly anxiety disorders, as well as premenstrual exacerbation of existing physical and mental health conditions.

Research on anxiety sensitivity and menstrual cycle reactivity indicates that women who report high levels of anxiety sensitivity also report increased levels of premenstrual distress (Sigmon et al., 2000). Furthermore, research suggests that the relationship between anxiety sensitivity and premenstrual symptoms may be impacted by the use of maladaptive coping strategies that exacerbate distress (Sigmon, Whitcomb-Smith, Rohan, & Kendrew, 2004). A recent review of the interaction between anxiety sensitivity and premenstrual symptoms in women with anxiety disorders suggested that high anxiety sensitivity and premenstrual hormone changes may result in clinical levels of anxiety when triggered by an external stressor (Nillni, Toufexis, & Rohan, 2011). This hypothesis is supported by research indicating that women reporting higher levels of premenstrual distress endorsed higher levels of self-reported panic following a panicogenic stress task (i.e., carbon dioxide challenge; Nillni, Rohan, Bernstein, & Zvolensky, 2010). In summary, previous research supports the influence of anxiety sensitivity in women's reports of premenstrual distress, implicating this construct as a potential vulnerability factor in premenstrual disorders.

Rumination, a form of depressive self-focus, has also been conceptualized as a type of self-focused attention. Rumination is a process of passive, inward-focused thoughts and behaviors related to depressed mood and the causes and consequences of depressed mood (Nolen-Hoeksema, 1998). Rumination can be maladaptive because it primes individuals to experience additional negative thoughts and memories, impairs problem solving, interferes with instrumental behaviors thus preventing positive reinforcement (Nolen-Hoeksema, 1998, and erodes social support (Nolen-Hoeksema, Wisco, & Lyubomirsky, 2008). Laboratory and naturalistic studies support the role of rumination in depression, and this construct has also been used to explain why significantly more women than men experience depression (Nolen-Hoeksema, 1991; Nolen-Hoeksema, 1998). Individuals with a ruminative response style may also be more reactive to stressors, and report increased negative affect in response to stressors compared to individuals who do not ruminate (Feldner, Leen-Feldner, Zvolensky, & Lejuez, 2006; Vickers & Vogeltanz-Holm, 2003). Therefore, one possibility is that women with premenstrual disorders tend to have a ruminative response style, and engage in rumination in reaction to premenstrual mood symptoms, thus exacerbating the symptoms.

Research has also supported the role of rumination in Seasonal Affective Disorder (SAD). Young and colleagues (1991) proposed the Dual Vulnerability Hypothesis (DVH), which suggests that individuals with SAD have two vulnerabilities to develop the disorder: a vulnerability to develop seasonal vegetative symptoms, and a vulnerability to develop cognitive/affective symptoms of depression in the context of, or in response to, those symptoms. Not everyone who experiences seasonal vegetative symptoms goes on to develop a seasonal mood episode, and research implicates rumination as a moderator between these two symptom groups (Young, Reardon, & Azam, 2008). The concept behind this model, suggesting that the manner in which individuals with SAD interpret and react to their symptoms can predict who develops SAD, could also be applied to premenstrual distress. PMS/PMDD may be etiologically similar to SAD, which is fitting given that both disorders are cyclical in nature and both involve a combination of physical and psychological symptoms. The results of one study suggest that rumination partially mediates the relationship between anxiety sensitivity and premenstrual distress (Sigmon, Schartel, Hermann, Cassel, & Thorpe, 2009), providing initial support for this idea.

In consideration of the established relationship between rumination and anxiety sensitivity with mood and anxiety disorders, and the high comorbidity rates between premenstrual disorders with mood and anxiety disorders, it follows that there may be a connection between these underlying constructs and PMS/PMDD. Anxiety sensitivity and rumination are two forms of self-focused attention that could account for the timing of menstrual-cycle related symptoms, high comorbidity rates, premenstrual exacerbation of other conditions, and why specific biological explanations have resulted in mixed research evidence.

Research indicates that changes associated with the menstrual cycle are common (Clayton, 2008) and no consistent differences have been found in hormone or neurotransmitter levels in women with PMS/PMDD compared to controls (e.g., Di Guilio & Reissing, 2006). It may be that there are no quantifiable biological differences in women with and without these disorders, but instead that some women may react to these changes differently. Alternately, biological causes for premenstrual disorders may be impacted considerably by psychological contributions. For example, some women may be more sensitive to hormone changes because they are more reactive to the physical and emotional changes that are associated with these changes. In this manner, the premenstrual phase of the menstrual cycle creates an opportunity for women to experience increased symptoms, and this may lead to women with the underlying vulnerability to respond to these types of symptoms using maladaptive coping strategies (e.g., forms of self-focused attention) leads to increased premenstrual distress. This model also helps explain why pharmacological treatments have been helpful for some, but not all, women with premenstrual disorders. Certain medications may help to regulate mood and/or hormone changes, and stabilization of these fluctuations may result in less opportunity respond to these changes in a maladaptive manner. This could help account for symptom improvement due to pharmacological intervention despite the lack of evidence for purely biological models of etiology.

Psychological Interventions

Pharmacological treatments for premenstrual disorders, including selective serotonin reuptake inhibitors (SSRIs), serotonergic tricyclic antidepressants, hormonal therapy, and oral contraceptive pills, have demonstrated efficacy in treating approximately 60% of women presenting with PMDD (Halbreich et al., 2006).

Pharmacological interventions, particularly SSRIs, are often regarded as first-line treatments for women with premenstrual disorders who have severe mood symptoms (Yonkers et al., 2008). However, many women do not benefit from these interventions. For example, a recent meta-analysis indicated that a higher percentage of women do *not* respond to SSRIs and oral contraceptive treatment compared to women who do respond (Halbreich, 2008). Given that a significant number of women do not receive benefit from pharmacological interventions, it is important that alternatives are explored, including psychological treatments. It is also possible that some women may prefer non-pharmacological treatments due to side-effects or contraindications (Lustyk et al., 2009), as well as differing personal preferences.

Based on the results of several published treatment trials, the only psychological treatment for premenstrual disorders with research support is cognitive-behavioral therapy (CBT; Blake, Salkovskis, Gath, Day, & Garrod, 1998; Hunter, 2003; Kirkby, 1994; Christensen & Oei, 1994). The cognitive-behavioral framework for PMDD suggests that women with premenstrual distress may be interpreting physiological changes in a negative way, and that modifying these negative cognitions women may improve their symptoms (Blake, 1995). The focus of CBT for PMDD is on the relationship between thoughts, feelings, and behavior, especially as they are related to the cyclical changes associated with the menstrual cycle. Women with premenstrual distress may be interpreting cyclic physiological changes (e.g., cramps, bloating, fatigue) in ways that exacerbate emotional reactions to them (Hunter, 2003). These assumptions may be learned though life experiences, as well as social and cultural values (Hunter, 2003). This framework is consistent with the potential role of self-focused attention and coping in premenstrual disorders, as discussed previously, given that focus on and negative interpretation of symptoms may increase distress.

Despite some promising findings, the state of the research at present is not sufficient to conclude that CBT is an empirically-supported intervention for premenstrual disorders. A recent review of treatments for PMS and PMDD concluded that studies on CBT have had methodological shortcomings, and have lacked statistically significant CBT intervention effects (Lustyk, Gerrish, Shaver, & Keys, 2009). However, these additional findings warrant additional controlled trials to establish whether CBT is effective for women with PMS and PMDD. An additional possible research avenue is the exploration of mindfulness and acceptance-based therapies in treatment of premenstrual disorders (Lustyk et al., 2009). Although it would be premature to interpret these findings as conclusive evidence for a psychologically-based etiology for premenstrual disorders, the results indicating CBT-related improvement in PMS/PMDD does provide some support that psychological factors may be involved in premenstrual disorders.

One possibility is that the current cognitive-behavioral approach and subsequent treatment to premenstrual disorders is limited because it does not specifically address the cyclical nature of physiological and affective changes in PMS and PMDD. Specifically, if self-focus on physical and psychological symptoms and maladaptive coping are related to the etiology of premenstrual disorders, treatment that explicitly addresses these tendencies could result in improved outcomes. For example, interoceptive exposure has demonstrated efficacy in the treatment of individuals with high anxiety sensitivity (Craske &

Barlow, 2008), and mindfulness and rumination-focused CBT (Watkins et al., 2007) have been shown to have benefit for decreasing rumination (Broderick, 2005). However, these treatments have not been investigated in women with premenstrual disorders. Additional research would be required to substantiate these hypotheses. This represents a promising new avenue of research.

Conclusion

In order to increase holistic understanding of women's health and provide adequate treatment, the interaction between menstrual cycle changes and psychological factors is an important area of research. Theoretical bases and empirical studies support the hypothesis that psychological contributions may help explain the etiology of premenstrual disorders. It is unlikely that any one etiological factor accounts for PMS and PMDD; however, the integration of biological, psychological, and social factors can provide a comprehensive understanding of these disorders that has significant implications for research and treatment.

References

Adewuya, A., Loto, P., & Adewumi, T. (2008). Premenstrual dysphoric disorder amongst Nigerian university students: prevalence, comorbid conditions, and correlates. *Archives of Women's Health, 11*(1), 13-18.

Allais, G., Gabellari, I., Burzio, C., Rolando, S., De Lorenzo, C., Mana, O., & Benedetto, C. (2012). Premenstrual syndrome and migraine. *Neurological Sciences, 33*(Suppl 1), S111-S115.

Andrzej, M., & Diana, J. (2006). Premenstrual syndrome: From etiology to treatment. *Maturitas, 55*(1), S47-S54.

American Psychiatric Association. (2000). *Diagnostic and statistical manual of mental disorders* (Revised 4th ed.). Washington, DC: Author.

Bailey, J. W., & Cohen, L. S. (1999). Prevalence of mood and anxiety disorders in women who seek treatment for premenstrual syndrome. *Journal of Women's Health & Gender-Based Medicine, 8*(9), 1181-1184.

Barnard, K., Frayne, S. M., Skinner, K. M., & Sullivan, L. M. (2003). Health status among women with menstrual symptoms. *Journal of Women's Health, 12*(9), 911-919.

Biggs, W. S., & Demuth, R. H. (2011). Premenstrual syndrome and premenstrual dysphoric disorder. American Family Physician, 84(7), 918-924.

Blake, F. (1995). Cognitive therapy for premenstrual syndrome. *Cognitive and Behavioral Practice, 2*, 167-185.

Blake, F., Salkovskis, P., Gath, D., Day, A., & Garrod, A. (1998). Cognitive therapy for premenstrual syndrome: A controlled trial. Journal of Psychosomatic Research, 45(4), 307-318.

Broderick, P. C. (2005). Mindfulness and coping with dysphoric mood: contrasts with rumination and distraction. *Cognitive therapy and research, 29*(5), 501-510.

Chawla, A., Swindle, R., Long, S., Kennedy, S., & Sterfield, B. (2002). Premenstrual dysphoric disorder: is there an economic burden of illness? *Medical Care, 40*, 1101-1112.

Christensen, A. P. & Oei, T. P. (1995). The efficacy of cognitive behavioral therapy in treating premenstrual dysphoric changes. *Journal of Affective Disorders, 33*, 57-63.

Clayton, A. (2008). Symptoms related to the menstrual cycle: diagnosis, prevalence, and treatment. *Journal of Psychiatric Practice, 14*(1), 13-21.

Cohen, L. S., Soares, C. N., Otto, M. W., Sweeney, B. H., Liberman, R. F., Harlow, B. L. (2002). Prevalence and predictors of premenstrual dysphoric disorder (PMDD) in older premenopausal women. *Journal of Affective Disorders, 70*, 125-132.

Cortina, S. (2005). Advancing women's health care: diagnostic, treatment, and social factors of PMDD. *Women & Therapy, 28*(2), 91-104.

Craske, M. G., & Barlow, D. H. (2008). Panic disorder and agoraphobia. In D. H. Barlow (Ed.) *Clinical Handbook of Psychological Disorders* (4th ed., pp.1-64). New York: The Guilford Press.

Cunningham, J., Yonkers, K. A., O'Brien, S., & Eriksson, E. (2009). Update on research and treatment of premenstrual dysphoric disorder. *Harvard Review of Psychiatry, 17*(2), 120-137.

Davis, L., & Yonkers, K. A. (1997). Diagnosis and treatment of premenstrual dysphoric disorder. *International Journal of Psychiatry in Clinical Practice, 1*, 149-156

Di Guilio, G., & Reissing, E. D. (2006). Premenstrual dysphoric disorder: prevalence, diagnosis considerations, and controversies. *Journal of Psychosomatic Obstetrics and Gynecology, 27*(4), 201-210.

Dorhofer, D. M., & Sigmon, S. T. (2002). Physiological and psychological reactivity in women with asthma: the effects of anxiety and menstrual cycle phase. *Behaviour Research and Therapy, 40*(1), 3-17.

Epperson, C. N., Steiner, M., Hartlage, S. A., Eriksson, E., Schmidt, P. J., Jones, I., & Yonkers, K. A. (2012). Premenstrual dysphoric disorder: evidence for a new category for DSM-5. *American Journal of Psychiatry, 169,* 465-475.

Feldner, M. T., Leen-Feldner, E. W., Zvolensky, M. J., Lejuez, C. W. (2006). Examining the associating between rumination, negative affectivity, and negative affect induced by a paced auditory serial addition task. *Journal of Behavior Therapy and Experimental Psychiatry, 37,* 171-187.

Fontana, A. M., & Badaway, S. Z. A. (1997). Perceptual and coping processes across the menstrual cycle: an investigation in premenstrual syndrome clinic and community sample. *Behavioral Medicine, 22*(4), 152-159.

Fornaro, M., & Perugi, G. (2010). The impact of premenstrual dysphoric disorder among 92 bipolar patients. *European Psychiatry, 25,* 450-454.

Forrester-Knauss C., Zemp S. E., Weiss, C., & Tschudin, S. (2011). The interrelation between premenstrual syndrome and major depression: results from a population-based sample. *BMC Public Health, 11,* 795.

Garcia-Esteve, L., Navarro, P., Ascaso, C., Torres, A., Aguado, J., Gelabert, E., & Martín-Santos, R. (2008). Family caregiver role and premenstrual syndrome as associated factors for postnatal depression. *Archives of Women's Mental Health, 11*(3), 193-200.

Gingnell, M., Comasco, E., Oreland, L., Fredrikson, M., & Sundström-Poromaa, I. (2010). Neuroticism-related personality traits are related to symptom severity in patients with premenstrual dysphoric disorder and to the serotonin transporter gene-linked polymorphism 5-HTTPLPR. *Archives of Women's Mental Health, 13*(5), 417-423.

Gladis, M. M., & Walsh, B. (1987). Premenstrual exacerbation of binge eating in bulimia. *The American Journal of Psychiatry, 144*(12), 1592-1595.

Gonda, X., Fountoulakis, K. N., Csukly, G., Telek, T., Pap, D., Rihmer, Z., & Bagdy, G. (2010). Association of a trait-like bias towards the perception of negative subjective life events with risk of developing premenstrual symptoms. *Progress in Neuro-Psychopharmacology & Biological Psychiatry, 34*(3), 500-505.

Halbreich U., O'Brien, P. M., Eriksson, E., Bäckström, T., Yonkers, K. A., & Freeman, E. W. (2006). Are there differential symptom profiles that improve in response to different pharmacological treatments of premenstrual syndrome/premenstrual dysphoric disorder? *CNS Drugs, 20*(7).

Halbreich, U. (2008). Selective serotonin reuptake inhibitors and initial oral contraceptives for the treatment of PMDD: effective but not enough. *CNS Spectrums, 13*(7), 566-572.

Halbreich, U., Borenestein, J., Pearlstein, T., & Kahn, L. (2003). The prevalence impairment, impact, and burden of premenstrual dysphoric disorder (PMS/PMDD). *Psychoneuroendocrinology, 28*, 1-23.

Hartlage, S., Arduino, K. E., & Gehlert, S. (2001). Premenstrual dysphoric disorder and risk for major depressive disorder: A preliminary study. *Journal of Clinical Psychology, 57*(12), 1571-1578.

Hartlage, S. A., & Gehlert, S. (2006). Differentiating premenstrual dysphoric disorder from premenstrual exacerbations of other disorders: a methods dilemma. *Clinical Psychology: Science and Practice, 8*(2), 242-253.

Hartlage, S. A., Freels, S., Gotman, N., & Yonkers, K. (2012). Criteria for premenstrual dysphoric disorder: secondary analyses of relevant data sets. *Archives of General Psychiatry, 69*(3), 300-305.

Herzog, A. G., Smithson, S. D., Fowler, K. M., Krishnamurthy, K. B., Sundstrom, D., Kalayjian, L. A., & ... Dworetzky, B. A. (2011). Premenstrual dysphoric disorder in women with epilepsy: Relationships to potential epileptic, antiepileptic drug, and reproductive endocrine factors. *Epilepsy & Behavior, 21*(4), 391-396.

Hourani, L. L., Yuan, H., & Bray, R. M. (2004). Psychosocial and lifestyle correlates of premenstrual symptoms among military women. *Journal of Women's Health, 13*(7), 812-821.

Hunter, M. (2003). Cognitive behavioral interventions for premenstrual and menopausal symptoms. *Journal of Reproductive and Infant Psychology, 21*(3),

Hsiao, M., Hsiao, C., & Liu, C. (2004). Premenstrual symptoms and premenstrual exacerbation in patients with psychiatric disorders. *Psychiatry and Clinical Neurosciences, 58*(2), 186-190.

Hylan, T. R., Sundell, K., & Judge, R. (1999). The impact of premenstrual symptomology on functioning and treatment-seeking behavior: Experience from the United States, United Kingdom, and France. *Journal of Women's Health & Gender, 8*(8), 1043-1052.

Ingram, R. E. (1990). Self-focused attention in clinical disorders: Review and a conceptual model. *Psychological Bulletin, 107*(2), 156-176.

Jahanfar, S., Lye, M. S., & Krishnarajah, I. S. (2011). The heritability of premenstrual syndrome. *Twin Research and Human Genetics, 14*(5), 433-436.

Kaspi, S. P., Otto, M. W., Pollack, M. H., Eppinger, S., & Rosenbaum, J. F. (1994). Premenstrual exacerbation of symptoms in women with panic disorder. *Journal of Anxiety Disorders, 8,* 131-138.

Kim, D. R., Gyulai, L. L., Freeman, E. W., Morrison, M. F., Baldassano, C. C., & Dubé, B. B. (2004). Premenstrual dysphoric disorder and psychiatric co-morbidity. *Archives of Women's Mental Health, 7*(1), 37-47.

Kirkby, R. J. (1994). Changes in premenstrual symptoms and irrational thinking following cognitive-behavioral coping skills training. *Journal of Consulting and Clinical Psychology, 62*(5), 1026-1032.

Klump, K. L., Keel, P. K., Culbert, K. M., & Edler, C. (2008). Ovarian hormones and binge eating: Exploring associations in community samples. *Psychological Medicine, 38*(12), 1749-1757.

Lustyk, M. K. B., Gerrish, W. G., Shaver, S., & Keys, S. L. (2009). Cognitive-behavioral therapy for premenstrual syndrome and premenstrual dysphoric disorder: a systematic review. *Archives of Women's Mental Health, 2009,* 12, 85-96.

McFarland, C., Ross, M., & DeCourville, N. (1989) Women's theories of menstruation and biases in recall of menstrual symptoms. *Journal of Personality and Social Psychology, 57*(3), 522-531.

McMillan, M., & Pihl, R. (1987). Premenstrual depression: a distinct entity. *Journal of Abnormal Psychology, 96,* 149-154.

Markens, S. (1996). The problematic of "experience": a political and cultural critique of PMS. *Gender and Society, 10*(1), 42-58.

Martignoni, E. E., Nappi, R. E., Citterio, A. A., Calandrella, D. D., Corengia, E. E., Fignon, A. A., & ... Nappi, G. G. (2002). Parkinson's disease and reproductive life events. *Neurological Sciences, 23*(Suppl2), S85-S86.

Mitchell, L.L., & Mitchell, C.W. (1998). Effects of premenstrual syndrome on coping style. *Psychology, 35*(1), 2-10.

Mor, N., & Winquist, J. (2002). Self-focused attention and negative affect: A meta-analysis. *Psychological Bulletin, 128*(4), 638-662.

National Center for Chronic Disease Prevention and Health Promotion (2012). *Morbidity and mortality weekly report (MMWR), 60*(51), 1747. Available from: http://www.cdc.gov/mmwr/preview/mmwrhtml/mm6051a7.htm

Nillni, Y. I., Rohan, K. J., Bernstein, A., & Zvolensky, M. J. (2010). Premenstrual distress predicts panic-relevant responding to a CO_2

challenge task among young adult females. *Journal of Anxiety Disorders, 24*, 416-422.

Nillni, Y. I., Toufexis, D. J., & Rohan, K. J. (2011). Anxiety sensitivity, the menstrual cycle, and panic disorder: a putative neuroendocrine and psychological interaction. *Clinical Psychology Review, 31*, 1183-1191.

Nolen-Hoeksema, S. (1991). Responses to depression and their effects on the duration of depressive episodes. *Journal of Abnormal Psychology, 100*(4), 569-582.

Nolen-Hoeksema, S. (1998). Ruminative coping with depression. In J. Heckhausen & C. Dweck (Eds.) *Motivation and Self-Regulation Across the Life Span.* Cambridge: Cambridge University Press.

Nolen-Hoeksema, S., Wisco, B. E., & Lyubomirsky, S. (2008). Rethinking rumination. *Perspectives on Psychological Science, 3*(5), 400-424.

O'Brien, P. M. S, Backstrom, T., Brown, C., Dennerstein, L., Endicott, J., Epperson, C., …, Yonkers, K. (2011). Towards a consensus on diagnostic criteria, measurement, and trial design of the premenstrual disorders: the ISPMD Montreal consensus. *Archives of Women's Mental Health, 14*, 13-21.

Payne, J. L., Roy, P. S., Murphy-Eberenz, K., Weismann, M., Swartz, K. L., McInnis, M. G., & … Potash, J. B. (2007). Reproductive cycle-associated mood symptoms in women with major depression and bipolar disorder. *Journal of Affective Disorders, 99*(1-3), 221-229.

Pearlstein, T. (2010). Premenstrual dysphoric disorder: out of the appendix. *Archives of Women's Mental Health, 13*, 21-23.

Pearlstein, T. B., Halbreich, U., Batzar, E. D., Brown, C. S., Endicott, J., Frank, E., & … Yonkers, K. A. (2000). Psychosocial functioning in women with premenstrual dysphoric disorder before and after treatment with sertraline or placebo. *Journal of Clinical Psychiatry, 61*(2), 101-109.

Pearlstein, T., Yonkers, K. A., Fayyad, R., & Gillespie, J. A. (2005). Pretreatment pattern of symptom expression in premenstrual dysphoric disorder. *Journal of Affective Disorders, 85*, 275-282.

Pilver, C. E., Kasl, S., Desai, R., & Levy, B. R. (2011). Exposure to American culture is associated with premenstrual dysphoric disorder among ethnic minority women. *Journal of Affective Disorders, 130*(1-2), 334-341.

Portella, A., Haaga, D. F., & Rohan, K. J. (2006). The association between seasonal and premenstrual symptoms is continuous and is not fully accounted for by depressive symptoms. *Journal of Nervous and Mental Disease, 194*(11), 833-837.

Resnick, A., Perry, W., Parry, B., Mostofi, N., & Udell, C. (1998). Neuropsychological performance across the menstrual cycle in women with and without premenstrual dysphoric disorder. *Psychiatry Research, 77*(3), 147-158.

Robinson, R. L., & Swindle, R. W. (2000). Premenstrual symptom severity: Impact on social functioning and treatment-seeking behaviors. *Journal of Women's Health & Gender-Based Medicine, 9*(7), 757-768.

Rubinow, D. R., Smith, M. J., Schenkel, L. A., Schmidt, P. J., & Dancer, K. (2007). Facial emotion discrimination across the menstrual cycle in owmen with premenstrual dysphoric disorder. *Journal of Affective Disorders, 108*, 87-94.

Schmidt, N. B., Lerew, D. R., & Trakowski, J. H. (1997). Body vigilance in panic disorder: evaluating attention to bodily perturbations. *Journal of Consulting and Clinical Psychology, 65*(2), 214-220.

Seeman, M. V. (2012). Menstrual exacerbation of schizophrenia symptoms. *Acta Psychiatrica Scandinavica, 125*(5), 363-371.

Sigmon, S. T., Craner, J. R., Yoon, K. L., & Thorpe, G. L. (2012). Premenstrual syndrome. In V.S. Ramachandran (Ed.). *Encyclopedia of Human Behavior* (pp. 167-173). New York, NY: Elsevier.

Sigmon, S., Rohan, K., Boulard, N., Dorhofer, D., & Whitcomb, S. (2000). Menstrual reactivity: the role of gender-specificity, anxiety sensitivity, and somatic concerns in self-reported menstrual distress. *Sex Roles, 43*(3-4), 143-161.

Sigmon, S. T., Schartel, J. G., Hermann, B. A., Cassel, A. G., & Thorpe, G. L. (2009). The relationship between premenstrual distress and anxiety sensitivity: the mediating role of rumination. *Journal of Rational-Emotive Cognitive-Behavior Therapy, 27*, 188-200.

Sigmon, S. T., Whitcomb-Smith, S. R., Rohan, K. J., & Kendrew, J. J. (2004). The role of anxiety level, coping styles, and cycle phase in menstrual distress. *Anxiety Disorders, 18*, 177-191.

Steiner, M., Peer, M., Palova, E., Freeman, E. W., Macdougall, M., & Soares, C. N. (2011). The premenstrual symptoms screening tool revised for adolescents (PSST-A): prevalence of severe PMS and premenstrual dysphoric disorder in adolescents. *Archives of Women's Mental Health, 14*, 77-81.

Takeda, T., Tasaka, K., Sakata, M., & Murata, Y. (2006). Prevalence of premenstrual syndrome and premenstrual dysphoric disorder in Japanese women. *Archives of Women's Mental Health, 9*(4), 209-212.

Tschudin, S., Bertea, P., & Zemp, E. (2010). Prevalence and predictors of premenstrual syndrome and premenstrual dysphoric disorder in a population-based sample. *Archives of Women's Mental Health, 13*(6), 485-494.

Veeninga, A. T., de Ruiter, C., & Kraaimaat, F. W. (1994). The relationship between late luteal phase dysphoric disorder and anxiety disorders. *Journal of Anxiety Disorders, 8(*3), 207-215.

Vickers, K. S., & Vogeltanz-Holm, N. D. (2003). The effects of rumination and distraction tasks on psychophysiological responses and mood in dysphoric and nondysphoric individuals. *Cognitive Therapy and Research, 27*(3), 331-348.

Vickers, K., & McNally, R. (2004). Is premenstrual dysphoria a variant of panic disorder?: a review. *Clinical Psychology Review, 24*(8), 933-956.

Watkins, E., Scott, J., Wingrove, J., Rimes, K., Bathurst, N., Steiner, H., Kennel-Webb, S., ... Malliaris, Y. (2007). Rumination-focused cognitive behaviour therapy for residual depression: a case series. *Behaviour Research and Therapy, 45*, 2144-2154.

World Health Organization (2001). Mental health: new understanding, new hope. *World Health Organization.* Retrieved from: http://www.who.int/whr/2001/en/index.html

Wittchen, H. Becker, E., Lieb, R., & Krause, P. (2002). Prevalence, incidence and stability of premenstrual dysphoric disorder in the community. *Psychological Medicine, 32*(1), 119-132.

Wittchen, H., Perkonigg, A. A., & Pfister, H. H. (2003). Trauma and PTSD - An overlooked pathogenic pathway for Premenstrual Dysphoric Disorder? *Archives of Women's Mental Health, 6*(4), 293-297.

Yang, M., Wallenstein, G., Hagan, M., Guo, A., Chang, J., & Kornstein, S. (2008). Burden of Premenstrual Dysphoric Disorder on Health-Related Quality of Life. *Journal of Women's Health, 17*(1), 113-121.

Yonkers, K., O'Brien, P., & Eriksson, E. (2008). Premenstrual syndrome. *Lancet, 371,* 1200-1210.

Yonkers, K. A., Pearlstein, T., & Rosenheck, R. A. (2003). Premenstrual disorders: Bridging research and clinical reality. *Archives of Women's Mental Health, 6,* 287-292.

Yonkers, K., O'Brien, P., & Eriksson, E. (2008). Premenstrual syndrome. *Lancet, 371,* 1200-1210.

Young, M. A., Watel, L. G., Lahmeyer, H. Q., & Eastman, C. I. (1991). The temporal onset of individual symptoms in winter depression:

differentiating underlying mechanisms. *Journal of Affective Disorders, 22*(4), 191-197.

Young, M. A., Reardon, A., & Azam, O. (2008). Rumination and vegetative symptoms: a test of the dual vulnerability model of seasonal depression. *Cognitive Therapy Research, 32*, 567-576.

In: Menstrual Cycle
Editor: Madeleine Gosselin

ISBN: 978-1-62417-945-7
© 2013 Nova Science Publishers, Inc.

Chapter IV

Effects of Female Sex Hormones on Appetite and Food Intake

Sonia A. Tucci*

School of Psychology, University of Liverpool,
Liverpool, United Kingdom

Abstract

This chapter aims to review the mechanisms underlying the fluctuations on appetite and food intake that occur during the female reproductive cycle. These changes are the consequence of sex hormones variations during the menstrual cycle,cycle; therefore the effect of externally administered hormones will be extensively addressed. Estradiol has been deemed as the main hormone responsible for the reduction of intake during the periovulatory period. Activation of nuclear oestrogen receptors in brain areas such as the hypothalamus, hindbrain and reward system seem to be behind these effects. In addition estradiol also seems to increase the satiating potency of peripheral anorexigenic signals which leads to an early termination of meals. During the pre menstrual phase of the cycle intake is increased and although the

* Corresponding author: Dr Sonia Tucci; School of Psychology; University of Liverpool; Eleanor Rathbone Building; Bedford Street South; Liverpool; L37 2LE; United Kingdom; Telephone: +44 1517941121; Fax: + 44 151 7946937; Email: sonia.tucci@liv.ac.uk; Additional email: sonia.tucci@gmail.com.

underlying mechanisms are still not totally clarified, they point toward progesterone mediated antagonism of estradiol's effects. Externally administered sex hormones are the most common method used for birth control; they are also employed as hormone replacement therapy after the menopause and for medical purposes such as the treatment of menstrual disorders and endometriosis. In general these hormones are well tolerated; however, concerns about weight gain are amongst the main reasons given for the rejection or suspension of the treatment. Although this effect is commonly reported the evidence supporting this assertion is controversial. This review aims to provide a summary of the findings up to date on the effects of contraceptives on appetite and intake.

Keywords: estradiol, oestrogens, progesterone, cravings, luteal, follicular, cholecystokinin, satiety, meals, neuroimaging, contraceptives

Abbreviations

AgRP	Agouti related peptide
CCK	Cholecystokinin
CNS	Central nervous system
COC	Combined oral contraceptives
ER	Oestrogen receptor
FSH	Follicle stimulating hormone
LH	Luteinising hormone
NPY	Neuropeptide Y
OC	Oral contraceptives
OVX	Ovariectomised
PMS	Premenstrual syndrome
PVN	Paraventricular nucleus
SHBG	Sex-hormone binding globulin
VMH	Ventromedial hypothalamus

Introduction

Human menstrual cycle averages 28 days and is divided into two main phases with day 1 as the day of menstruation onset. The follicular phase starts on day one and ends with ovulation (day 14-15) whereas the luteal phase starts when ovulation takes place and lasts until the onset of the next menstruation (Owen, 1975).

The menstrual cycle arises as a consequence of the hormonal fluctuations of the ovarian cycle which in turn is controlled by hypothalamic hormones. The follicular phase is characterised by a progressive increase in oestrogen levels which feedback positively on luteinising hormone (LH). On day 14 a LH peak induces ovulation and if no fertilisation takes place oestrogen levels drop within 24 hours.

After ovulation, LH triggers the transformation of the follicle granulosa cells into progesterone-producing cells (corpus luteum), leading to elevated progesterone levels throughout the luteal phase.

If no implantation occurs, progesterone levels will drop after 14 days which leadleading to the shedding of the endometrium (Channing, Schaerf, Anderson, and Tsafriri, 1980).

Although this cycle is present and somehow similar in most mammalian placental females, the immediate post-ovulatory phase tends to be species specific. In this chapter, the ovarian cycle of the rat will be briefly reviewed since most pre clinical studies that have investigated the effects of sex hormones on intake have been carried out in this species. Contrary to primates, rodents do not shed the endometrium at the end of the cycle, instead, they reabsorb it.

Thus rats' oestrous cycle is the equivalent of the primate menstrual cycle and it lasts 4-5 days. It comprises four phases: proestrus, oestrus, metoestrus (or dioestrus I) and dioestrus (or dioestrus II). Ovulation takes place from the beginning of proestrus to the end of oestrus. In terms of hormonal changes, in the afternoon of the proestrus phase there is an increase of both (LH) and follicle stimulating hormone (FSH).

This is followed by an increase of estradiol which reaches peak levels in proestrus and returns to baseline at oestrus. Progesterone secretion peaks twice, during metoestrus and dioestrus and at the end of proestrus (Freeman, 1988).

Rats do not experience the post ovulatory increase of oestrogen and progesterone found in women. However, both humans and rodents share the decrease of FSH and LH secretion that takes place in the final phase of the cycle. In terms of food intake, rodents also experience a variation across the oestrous cycle being at its maximum in dioestrus, followed by proestrus, with the smallest intake observed in oestrus (Eckel, 1999). It is important to note that the differences in the post ovulatory phase of the cycle make rodents poor models to study appetite regulation and food intake in this phase of the cycle (Asarian and Geary, 2006).

Oestrogen Modulation of Food Intake

Estrone, estradiol, and estriol are the primary female sex hormones in vertebrates and constitute the three major naturally occurring oestrogens. Estradiol is the predominant oestrogen in non pregnant females from menarche to menopause.

Estradiol influences body composition by both altering appetite and intake and also affecting metabolic parameters such as protein synthesis (Price et al., 1998) and energy expenditure (Richard, 1986). However, it seems to be generally agreed that the main effect of estradiol is on intake with minor alterations of metabolic rate (Bisdee, James, and Shaw, 1989).

Intake is inhibited by oestrogens in both a tonic and cyclic fashion. The tonic inhibitory effect is constant throughout the cycle and it is evidenced by a decrease of intake during the reproductive ages when compared with post menopausal years. The decrease of oestrogen levels during the menopause or in ovariectomised (OVX) rats correlates with an increase on intake and adiposity. The cyclic inhibitory effect occurs during the peri-ovulatory phase where estradiol is at its peak (Asarian and Geary, 2006). Oestrogens seem to advance the onset of satiety decreasing in consequence the size of the meals (Eckel, 1999). On average food intake is 10% lower during the follicular phase with no fluctuation seen in anovulatory cycles (Pelkman, Heinbach, and Rolls, 2000). This effect is mirrored in rats and mice where there is a decrease of 25% on intake on the night that follows ovulation which coincides with an oestrogen peak.

It has been proposed that oestrogens regulate feeding by several mechanisms which involve direct effects through stimulation of oestrogen receptors in the central nervous system (CNS) and also indirect effects on peripheral signals.

Role of Oestrogen Receptors

In the CNS estradiol exerts many of its actions by coupling with the nuclear oestrogen receptors ERα and ERβ. ERα are predominantly found in the hypothalamus, while ERβ have a wider distribution (Shughrue, Lane, and

Merchenthaler, 1997). Both receptors are known to participate in intake regulation (Liang et al., 2002). OVX mice with a null mutation of ERα do not decrease their intake in response to estradiol administration suggesting that at least in part, ERα mediate estradiol's anorectic actions (Geary, Asarian, Korach, Pfaff, and Ogawa, 2001). Furthermore, administration of the ERα agonist propyl-pyrazole-triol induces both chronic and acute suppression of intake in OVX rats (Roesch, 2006). ERβ also modulate estradiol's effects on intake. For instance, estradiol's anorexigenic effects can be blocked with anti-sense oligodeoxynucleotides for ERβ (Liang et al., 2002).

In addition, administration of estradiol into the paraventricular nucleus of the hypothalamus (PVN) reduces intake, and in this area oestrogen sensitive neurones only express ERβ (Shughrue et al., 1997). Furthermore, in OVX rats selective blockade of ERα expression in the ventromedial hypothalamus (VMH) does not attenuate the effect of systemic estradiol (Musatov et al., 2007). Apart from its direct involvement on intake, it has been suggested that ERβ also modulate the hedonic aspects of eating since they have been found in reward system regions such as the striatum and nucleus accumbens (Creutz and Kritzer, 2002). Furthermore, OVX reduces dopamine binding in these areas (Le Saux, Morissette, and Di Paolo, 2006) hindering dopamine reward signalling which in turn could lead to a compensatory increase in food consumption. Thus oestrogen signalling at ERβ could be relevant to hedonic eating.

Central Effects of Oestrogen

Although the main effects of estradiol on food intake seem to be mediated through actions on peripheral signals, some experimental evidence points towards additional direct actions on the CNS. Early studies found that administration of estradiol to the VMH of OVX rats decreased intake. It was suggested that one mechanism by which estradiol decreased food intake was by altering the body weight set point in the VMH (Jankowiak and Stern, 1974).

More recently it has been proposed that estradiol alters the expression of hypothalamic neuropeptides involved in feeding behaviour (Olofsson, Pierce, and Xu, 2009). Neuropeptide Y (NPY)/Agouti related peptide (AgRP) neurones have been identified as crucial targets. To date, NPY is one of the most potent orexigenic signals known whereas AgRP increases food intake by acting as an antagonist at melanocortin receptors. Agonism at melanocortin receptors reduces food intake therefore its blockade would increase it (Morton and Schwartz, 2001). In mice the elimination of AgRP neurones abolished the oestrous cycle dependent changes in feeding and body weight (Olofsson et al., 2009). Moreover, the expression of NPY and AgRP is down-regulated by estradiol and their mRNA production is increased by OVX (Titolo, Cai, and Belsham, 2006). Estradiol also modulates the sensitivity to exogenous NPY since its administration decreases NPY's orexigenic effects and inhibits the activity of NPY/AgRP neurones in the arcuate nucleus of the hypothalamus.

Peripheral Effects of Oestrogen

Ghrelin

Ghrelin is a peptide hormone secreted by the stomach which increases food intake (Kojima et al., 1999). Oestrogens seem to modulate the effects of ghrelin. For instance, oestrogen administration to OVX rats attenuates the orexigenic effects of exogenous ghrelin. It has been suggested that estradiol exerts a tonic inhibitory effect on ghrelin receptors (Clegg et al., 2007). The effects of estradiol on ghrelin secretion have not been fully elucidated. Some studies have found that oestrogens decrease ghrelin secretion (Clegg et al., 2007) whilst others found no effects (Dafopoulos, Sourlas, Kallitsaris, Pournaras, and Messinis, 2009).

Cholecystokinin (CCK)

CCK is a gastrointestinal hormone that amongst other functions,functions has an important role in the onset of satiation (Smith and Gibbs, 1992). In rats CCK mediates oestrogen's peri-ovulatory decrease of intake. These effects are specific to certain brain areas, estradiol implants in the surface of the brainstem and PVN, but not other brain areas, potentiate the satiating action of peripheral CCK (Asarian and Geary, 2007). Thus, it seems that at least in rats, the main effect of estradiol is to increase the potency rather than the secretion of CCK (Butera, Bradway, and Cataldo, 1993). These effects vary across the ovarian cycle, CCK receptor antagonism produces a bigger de-satiating effect in oestrus (when estradiol levels are high) than in dioestrus (when estradiol levels are low) (Huang et al., 1993).

Leptin

Leptin is a hormone synthesised by the adipose tissue; its circulating levels mirror the total amount of body fat. In both humans and animals there is a positive correlation between leptin and oestrogen levels (Caro et al., 1996; Considine et al., 1996). Although it has been suggested that body weight moderates the interaction between oestrogen, leptin and food intake (Gambacciani et al., 1997), experimental evidence on the involvement of oestrogen in leptin signalling in not conclusive. Some studies report that estrogens increase leptin's anorexigenic actions (Clegg, Riedy, Smith, Benoit, and Woods, 2003) whilst others found no significant effects (Chung, Bond, and Jarrett, 2010; Pelleymounter, Baker, and McCaleb, 1999). These discrepancies could arise from methodological differences making this a topic that requires further investigation.

Progesterone

Administration of progesterone to intact rats increases appetite and body weight (Wade and Schneider, 1992). However, the effects of progesterone seem to be estradiol dependent since in OVX rats progesterone administered at physiological doses does not alter feeding behaviour (Butera, 2010; Davidsen, Vistisen, and Astrup, 2007). Furthermore, in these animals the anorexigenic effect of estradiol is prevented by co-administration of progesterone (Blaustein and Wade, 1976; Jankowiak and Stern, 1974; Wade, 1975). These findings have led to the suggestion that the increase on intake observed in luteal phase could be the result of progesterone antagonism of oestrogen's anorexigenic effects. However, further studies are required to examine this hypothesis (Davidsen et al., 2007).

Food Intake during the Menstrual Cycle

As mentioned above, in both menstruating women and laboratory animals, intake is lowest during the periovulatory phase of the ovarian cycle, when estradiol levels are high (Buffenstein, Poppitt, McDevitt, and Prentice, 1995). During the luteal phase there is an increase of intake that has been consistently seen in both self-reported (food diaries, interviews, measurement of food weight at home) (Barr, Janelle, and Prior, 1995; Dalvit, 1981; Danker-Hopfe, Roczen, and Löwenstein-Wagner, 1995; Lyons, Truswell, Mira, Vizzard, and Abraham, 1989 ; Martini, Lampe, Slavin, and Kurzer, 1994; Pliner and Fleming, 1983) and laboratory measurements (Tucci, Murphy, Boyland, Dye, and Halford, 2010; Tucci, Murphy, Boyland, and Halford, 2009; Tucci et al.,

2011). The daily increase on intake varies from around 150 kcal (7.5%) (Gong, Garrel, and Calloway, 1989; Martini et al., 1994; Pohle-Krauza, Carey, and Pelkman, 2008) to doubling the amount of intake when compared to the follicular phase (Lyons et al., 1989). However, it should be noted that not all studies have found clear effects of phase on total intake.

Nutrient Selection

In terms of estradiol's effects on nutrients choice, research has reported controversial results. Whilst some studies in rats have found that oestrous cycle impacts nutrient selection (Leibowitz, Akabayashi, Alexander, and Wang, 1998) others found no such effects (Geiselman, Martin, VanderWeele, and Novin, 1981). Similarly, in women findings are also contradictory with some reporting no cyclical effects on food selection (Cheikh Ismail, Al-Hourani, Lightowler, Aldhaheri, and Henry, 2009) whereas other have found some alterations. For instance, a study by Chung et al (Chung et al., 2010) found that the increased caloric intake observed during the luteal phase was almost exclusively due to an increase in protein intake. Others have reported that the increased caloric intake in this phase was due to an increased intake of fat (Johnson, Corrigan, Lemmon, Bergeron, and Crusco, 1994; Li, Tsang, and Lui, 1999) or carbohydrates (Dalvit-McPhillips, 1983).

Two studies performed in our laboratory found that at least for snack items, participants consumed more sweet snacks during luteal phase that follicular phase (Tucci et al., 2010; Tucci et al., 2011), these findings are consistent with previous reports regarding sweet food (Bowen and Grunberg, 1990) and chocolate consumption (Hetherington and MacDiarmid, 1993). In our study although participants consumed more calories derived from sweet items in the luteal phase, the ratings of liking for these foods did not increase when compared to the follicular phase. This disconnection between actual intake and a key element of feeding motivation appears somewhat puzzling. Therefore, these data support the more physiological notion that the phase based difference in snack food intake are largely consequence of weakened post-meal satiety rather than driven by altered food cravings and preferences.

Additionally, binge eating is also more likely to occur in the luteal phase (Klump, Keel, Culbert, and Edler, 2008). Binge eating has been associated with low levels of plasma and brain serotonin (Cross, Marley, Miles, and Willson, 2001). Moreover, women with premenstrual syndrome (PMS) have lower levels of serotonin and more episodes of binge eating when compared with their non-PMS counterparts (Rapkin et al., 1987). Low levels of serotonin contribute to the mood changes experienced during the premenstrual period which are more pronounced in PMS. Carbohydrate consumption can influence brain serotonin levels by increasing the ratio of tryptophan: large amino acids. Tryptophan, the precursor of serotonin, competes with large amino acids for entry into the brain. It has been proposed that the increase in carbohydrate consumption during binge eating is an attempt to elevate brain serotonin levels in order to improve mood. Both animal and human studies support the hypothesis that low levels of brain serotonin may play a role in binge eating (Rapkin et al., 1987).

Cravings

Food cravings are very prevalent, with almost all women and 75% of men reporting food or drink cravings at some point in their lives (Pelchat, 1997; Rodin, Mancuso, Granger, and Nelbach, 1991). There is a gender difference regarding the type of food craved, men crave savoury food while women crave sweet food, especially chocolate (Pelchat, 1997; Weingarten and Elston, 1991). Cravings vary across the menstrual cycle being more intense perimenstrually (Bruinsma and Taren, 1999; Zellner, Garriga-Trillo, Centeno, and Wadsworth, 2004). This periodicity has led to the idea that cravings for sweets (especially chocolate) are the result of some physiological adjustment (Bruinsma and Taren, 1999). Two explanations have been proposed, one suggests that in this period a need state is created which is satisfied by some ingredient in chocolate (e.g. magnesium or serotonin). The second suggestion is that chocolate contains some ingredient that causes pleasure, either directly or indirectly through neurotransmitter release (e.g. endogenous opioids), which for some unknown reason is desired more perimenstrually.

The physiological explanations of perimenstrual cravings are not fully supported. For instance no significant correlations between levels of oestrogen or progesterone and craving (mainly chocolate cravings) frequency and intensity throughout the cycle have been found (Rodin et al., 1991). In addition, if chocolate is given in capsules, which avoids identification, cravings are not satisfied (Michener, Rozin, Freeman, and Gale, 1999). Thus non-physiological causes of chocolate cravings seem to be more probable. This is further supported by the fact that cravings are significantly less frequent in Spanish (16.7%) than in American women (27.8%) (Zellner, Garriga-Trillo, Rohm, Centeno, and Parker, 1999).

The above findings have led to the suggestion that cravings could be the result of learned associations between the craving experience and times of the menstrual cycle characterised by unpleasant physical "symptoms" (Yonkers, O'Brien, and Eriksson, 2008). Therefore they could be the result of some learned strategy such as the perceptual properties of the chocolate and/or the fact that chocolate is viewed as a 'special treat' with specific perceptual properties (Dye, 2001). Others have proposed that cravings are the result of avoiding certain foods whose intake is restricted during the post ovulatory phase. Thus food restriction can lead to craving for the avoided foods, which are usually high fat items (Channon and Hayward, 1990). This theory is supported by a recent study which found a correlation between fear of fatness, strength of cyclical variation in hunger, food cravings and amount eaten (McVay, Copeland, and Geiselman, 2011). Three explanations are offered for these findings, one proposes that large cyclical variations in appetite and food intake result in concomitant variations in body weight which in turn increase concerns about body weight. A second explanation claims that fear of fatness could trigger cyclical fluctuations in appetite and other eating variables. An increased fear of fatness would lead to a perception that the fluctuations in hunger that occur as part of the menstrual cycle are a threat to an idealised body image. This in turn would intensify the focus on hunger, food cravings and food intake. Finally a third explanation suggests an underlying variable which is responsible for the association between fear of fatness and cyclical variations in eating.

Role of Endogenous Sex Hormones in the Development of Obesity

In both females and males, sex hormones have play an important role in the distribution of fat mass. The androgen to oestrogen ratio seems to be a key regulator of adipose tissue homeostasis and distribution. Alterations of this ratio lead to fat accumulation and consequently weight gain (Quarta, Mazza, Pasquali, and Pagotto, 2012). In both genders, a reduced conversion of androgens into oestrogens contributes to body weight gain and obesity-related metabolic complications (Jones et al., 2000). In wWomen with hyperandrogenism (as for the case of polycystic ovary syndrome) there is often have an increased of visceral fat (Gambineri et al., 2009). The increase in fat deposition is the result of an increased appetite and an altered fat metabolism. Hyperandrogenic women have altered appetite regulation (Hirschberg, Naessén, Stridsberg, Byström, and Holte, 2004) which in some cases is associated to bulimia. It has been suggested that high androgen levels might promote cravings, alter impulse control (Cotrufo et al., 2000; Sundblad, Landen, Eriksson, Bergman, and Eriksson, 2005) and decrease satiety., Tthis is supported by the finding that post meal CCK levels are lower in bulimics and normalised by the administration of antiandrogen medication (Naessén, Carlström, Byström, Pierre, and Hirschberg, 2007). Stressful events also seem to alter Tthe androgen to oestrogen ratio is also altered by stressful events, and thus these events can triggering the onset of abdominal obesity particularly in women (Torres and Nowson 2007). Stress increases the activity of the hypothalamic-pituitary axis with a consequent increase of circulating levels of cortisol, which in turn inhibits lipid mobilisation in adipocytes. Amongst the different types of body fat, visceral fat displays the highest density of cortisol receptors, therefore under stressful conditions,conditions; it would be these areas where fat deposition would be more accentuated (Bjorntorp and Rosmond, 2000).

The increased depots of visceral fat lead to insulin resistance and secondary hyperinsulinemia. Insulin increases circulating levels of testosterone by two mechanisms: stimulation of ovarian testosterone production and inhibition of sex-hormone binding globulin (SHBG) synthesis in the liver (Crave, Lejeune, Brebant, Baret, and Pugeat, 1995; Poretsky, 1991). In women raised testosterone levels trigger insulin resistance and accumulation of abdominal fat. Testosterone also has an inhibitory effect on SHBG production. (Michalakis, Mintziori, Kaprara, Tarlatzis, and Goulis, 2012). Conversely, in men increased abdominal fat deposits are associated with low levels of testosterone and weight loss increases testosterone levels and normalises insulin sensitivity (Mogri, Dhindsa, Quattrin, Ghanim, and Dandona, 2012).

Effects of Externally Administered Sex Hormones during Reproductive Ages

Female sex hormones are administered to women during fertile ages primarily to avoid pregnancies. However, they are also employed with other purposes such as the reduction in risk of endometrial carcinoma, iron deficiency anaemia and dysmenorrhoea.

In addition, their effects on the cervical mucus have also been proposed to be protective against pelvic inflammatory disease (Wanyonyi, Stones, and Sequeira, 2011). Hormonal contraceptives are amongst the most commonly used contraceptive methods (including both reversible and non-reversible methods). Of these oral contraceptives (OC) are the largest group. Worldwide they are used by 9% of women between the ages of 15 and 49 and in developed regions this figure raises to 18- 30% ("United Nations, Department of Economic and Social Affairs, Population Division. World Ccontraceptive use", 2011). OC include both combined oral contraceptives (COC: contain oestrogen and progestin) as well as progestin-only pills. Next in usage are injectables and implants. Some injectable contraceptives are combined, while others like depot medroxyprogesterone acetate (DMPA, depo provera®) are progestin-only. The advantage of injectables and implants is that they are long-acting, thus freeing women from daily action to prevent unintended pregnancy. Long-acting methods are among the most cost-effective contraceptives in many areas. The first COC (Enovid; Searle) was developed in 1960. It contained oestrogen and progestin which prevented pregnancy by inhibiting ovulation and implantation (Burkman, Bell, and Serfaty, 2011). Progestin prevents ovulation by decreasing LH levels. Although oestrogen contributes to this effect by suppressing both FSH and LH, it was originally added to COC mainly to provide better cycle control. Since their initial development, COC have undergone significant modifications that involved alterations of hormone types, doses and administration regimes.

The first pills contained oestrogen doses of 150 mcg, this has been reduced to around 35 mcg in the currently available ones. Although the oestrogen dose does not seem to alter contraceptive effectiveness, side effects such as increased risk of venous thromboembolism, bloating, breast tenderness and nausea seem to be dose dependent. Lowering the dose below 20 mcg produces bleeding irregularities (Gallo, Nanda, Grimes, Lopez, and Schulz, 2008).

Similarly to oestrogens, the progestin content of COC has also been reduced from 10 mg in the first pills to 0.5 -1.5 mg. In addition, several new progestins have been introduced, each differing in potency, affinity for the progesterone and other steroid receptors, interactions with oestrogen and physiological effects.

Many progestins are derived from testosterone, and therefore produce undesirable effects such as acne, hirsutism and altered carbohydrate metabolism (Sitruk-Ware, 2006). The wide range of COC formulations currently available are in general well tolerated, with few side-effects various side effects which in their majority are related to the suppression of ovarian estradiol production. Nonetheless, about half of hormonal contraceptives users discontinue within 1 year of their first prescription most often because of side-effects or concerns about adverse health effects (Mishell, 2004). Many women, especially adolescents, stop taking them because of weight gain, mood swings and sexual dissatisfaction (Westhoff et al., 2007).

Hormonal Contraceptives and Weight Gain

It is important to highlight that weight gain cannot be solely attributed to an increase in fat deposition, it can also be due to fluid retention and increase in muscle mass (lean mass). These factors must be taken into account when in studies reviewing the effects of hormonal contraceptive on weight. Fear of weight gain is deemed as one of the main issues that hinders the acceptance and maintenance of contraceptives use (Lindh, Blohm, Andersson-Ellström, and Milsom, 2009; Lindh, Ellström, and Milsom, 2011). For younger women, who are particularly aware of their body image, this aspect is of high relevance. Between 50 and 75% of women in reproductive ages believe that weight gain is associated with the use of OC (Oddens, 1999; Wysocki, 2000); and give this as the main reason for discontinuation (Rosenberg and Waugh, 1998). Importantly, this perception is shared by clinicians. A Canadian study reported that 68% of practitioners informed women who were prescribed OC that weight gain was a possible unwanted side effect (Gaudet, Kives, Hahn, and Reid, 2004).

Randomised clinical trials on this topic are rare due to the risk of unwanted pregnancies. The 2011 Cochrane review revealed no clear evidence of weight gain with the use of COC (Gallo, Lopez, Grimes, Schulz, and Helmerhorst, 2011). However, the studies analysed have methodological differences of which the most important is the control group used.

Factors such the tendency that individuals have to gain weight over time (Flegal and Troiano, 2000) should be taken into account and in absence of a reliable control group, a definition of what is regarded as excessive weight gain is needed and no consensus about it has been reached.

COC use in adolescent girls in developed countries is approximately 50% (Lara-Torre, 2009). An extensive review performed by Warholm et al. (Warholm, Petersen, and Ravn, 2012) reported that the majority of studies found no evidence of weight gain caused by COC in this age group. However, although weight gain is not significant it is still accounted by users as the most common secondary effect.

The apparent weight gain reported could be due to several factors, firstly, self reported measures of weight gain do not tend to coincide with measurements taken in the laboratory. Girls tend to report a much bigger weight gain that the one measured which confirms the misconception that prevails among users. Secondly, in this age group normal weight gain it is expected due to growth. Similarly to the effects of COC on weight gain, reports investigating the effects of DMPA on body weight have also reported equivocal results. An early study by Amatayakul (Amatayakul, Sivasomboon, and Thanangkul, 1980) reported that DMPA increased fat deposition whereas a study by Pelkman et al. (Pelkman et al., 2000) found no effects on weight or appetite. The studies that suggest that DMPA alters weight report a huge variability: −5 kg to +12 kg at 12 months (Risser, Gefter, Barratt, and Risser, 1999) and −25 lbs to + 69 lbs at 6 months (Leiman, 1972).

This variability is attributed to different characteristics of the population receiving the contraceptive. For instance, DMPA seems to have different effects on weight gain depending on several factors.

A longitudinal study by Le and colleagues (Le, Rahman, and Berenson, 2009) identified several risk factors for early weigh gain (body mass index (BMI) < 30, parity of 1 or more,more and self-reported increase of appetite). In turn, early weight gain is a predictor of further weight gain. In addition age seems to have an influence, obese adolescents appear to be at higher risk of gaining weight when receiving DMPA than non obese ones (Bonny, Ziegler, and Harvey, 2006), whereas in older women lower initial BMI's seem to predict bigger weight gains (Le et al., 2009).

DMPA effects on appetite also seem to be modulated by race, in black adolescent DMPA decreases appetite whilst it increases it in their white counterparts (Bonny et al., 2006). It can be concluded that the effects of DMPA on appetite and weight gain seem to be modulated by the interaction of several factors that should be taken into account when prescribing these contraceptives.

Hormonal Contraceptives Appetite and Food Intake

Similarly to the effects of COC on body weight, studies that investigated their effects on appetite and food intake have reported contradictory results. Some have reported that COC increase intake (Eck et al., 1997; Naessén, Carlström, Byström, Pierre, and Hirschberg, 2007) whereas others found no effects (Massé, 1991; McNeill, Bruce, Ross, and James, 1988; Procter-Gray et al., 2008).

These ambiguous results could be in part due to methodological flaws, for instance, the use of self-report dietary records or interviews (Eck et al., 1997; Wallace, Heiss, Burrows, and Graves, 1987) is affected by the strong bias towards under-reporting habitual energy intake (Black et al., 1991).

Fewer studies have employed methods where food intake is measured directly by weighing food before and after a meal (Naessén et al., 2007; Tucci et al., 2010; Tucci et al., 2011). The results of a study performed in our laboratory showed that COC use reverses the patterns observed during a regular menstrual cycle where intake is increased in the luteal phase. COC users consumed more food in the follicular phase. However, it is important to note that the total caloric intake across one cycle when comparing OC users and not users was similar.

The results of this study allow proposing that COC seem to reverse the cycling fluctuations in intake observed during the menstrual cycle. COC increased intake at the beginning of the pill cycle which might compensate for the decreased intake during the luteal phase equivalent. (Tucci et al., 2011).

In terms of macronutrient selections the findings are similar; some report that COC modifies selection whilst others found no effects. The study by Eck and colleagues (Eck et al., 1997) found that COC users consumed a greater percentage of energy as fat, and a lesser percentage of energy as carbohydrates when compared with non users.

Our study found that although COC did not alter macronutrient selection, users consumed more high fat sweet items. This effect was independent of the cycle phase. COC also seems to have an effect on cravings. Bancroft and Rennie (Bancroft and Rennie, 1993) reported a non significant trend towards craving for sweets during the hormone free week (withdrawal bleeding).

Naessen and colleagues found that OC increased cravings for fats (Naessén et al., 2007). A suppression of postprandial CCK release has been proposed as one mechanism by which COC increase intake (Hirschberg, Bystrom, Carlstrom, and von Schoultz, 1996; Karlsson, Linden, and von Schoultz, 1992).

This would lead to a decrease post-meal satiety and snacking. Progestins are known to stimulate food intake (Maltoni et al., 2001). They have been used to treat cancer-related cachexia and anorexia and other forms of malnutrition. They increase insulin levels and decrease CCK secretion (Karlsson et al., 1992) which would ultimately lead to weight gain. In contrast antiandrogenic OC containing ethinylestradiol and drospirenone attenuate binge eating and reduce appetite (Naessén et al., 2007).

Users of contraceptives with this particular composition seem to experience a small reduction in body weight (Sitruk-Ware, 2006). However, despite extensive clinical experience with OC treatment, little is presently known concerning the effects of different types of OC on appetite and body weight and much more research in this area is clearly necessary.

Conclusion

The fluctuations of sex hormones produced by the ovarian cycle are responsible for the variations on appetite and intake that have been consistently found in human and animal females. Estradiol reduces intake by acting on central and peripheral signals that regulate intake. Both oestrogen receptors are responsible of estradiol's anorexigenic effects. In the CNS oestrogens decrease the activity of hypothalamic orexigenic signals such as NPY and AgRP. In addition, estradiol modulates the brain sensitivity to peripheral satiety signals such as CCK. Although progesterone on its own does not seem to modify intake, in the luteal phase, when its levels are increased it seems to antagonise oestrogen's anorexigenic actions. This has been proposed as the mechanism behind the increased intake observed in the luteal phase. In terms of nutrient selection, the findings are inconclusive with some reporting a luteal non specific increase in intake and others reporting specific increases of proteins, fats or carbohydrates intake. The majority thus agrees that carbohydrates tend to be the most craved and over consumed items and during this phase. Pathological alterations of sex hormones levels have been associated with some types of eating disorders and obesity. Furthermore, one of the most commonly reported side effects and reason for discontinuation hormonal contraception is weight gain. This review attempted to summarise the findings regarding this issue.

To date the evidence supporting the belief that hormonal contraceptives increase weight is weak if not nonexistent. However, it is important to note that it is very difficult to generate assertive conclusions due to the fact that studies of this type face important methodological constraints such as the lack of a valid control group and the amount of variables (race, age, baseline BMI, different OC dosages, and parity) that influence the results.

References

Amatayakul, K., Sivasomboon, B., and Thanangkul, O. (1980). A study of the mechanism of weight gain in medroxyprogesterone acetate users. *Contraception, 22*(6), 605-622.

Asarian, L., and Geary, N. (2006). Modulation of appetite by gonadal steroid hormones. *Philos. Trans R Soc. Lond B Biol. Sci., 361*, 1251-1263.

Asarian, L., and Geary, N. (2007). Estradiol enhances cholecystokinin-dependent lipid-induced satiation and activates estrogen receptor-alpha-expressing cells in the nucleus tractus solitarius of ovariectomized rats. *Endocrinology, 148*(12), 5656-5666.

Bancroft, J., and Rennie, D. (1993). The impact of oral contraceptives on the experience of perimenstrual mood, clumsiness, food craving and other symptoms. *J. Psychosom. Res., 37*(2), 195-202.

Barr, S. I., Janelle, K. C., and Prior, J. C. (1995). Energy intakes are higher during the luteal phase of ovulatory menstrual cycles. *Am. J. Clin. Nutr., 61*(1), 39-43.

Bisdee, J. T., James, W. P., and Shaw, M. A. (1989). Changes in energy expenditure during the menstrual cycle. *Br. J. Nutr., 61*(2), 187-199.

Bjorntorp, P., and Rosmond, R. (2000). Obesity and cortisol. *Nutrition, 16*, 924-936.

Black, A. E., Goldberg, G. R., Jebb, S. A., Livingstone, M. B., Cole, T. J., and Prentice, A. M. (1991). Critical evaluation of energy intake data using fundamental principles of energy physiology: 2. Evaluating the results of published surveys. *Eur. J. Clin. Nutr., 45*(12), 583-599.

Blaustein, J. D., and Wade, G. N. (1976). Ovarian influences on the meal patterns of female rats. *Physiol. Behav., 17*(2), 201-208.

Bonny, A. E., Ziegler, J., and Harvey, R. (2006). Weight gain in obese and nonobese adolescent girls initiating depot medroxyprogesterone, oral contraceptive pills, or no hormonal contraceptive method. *Arch. Pediatr. Adolesc. Med., 160*, 40-45.

Bowen, D. J., and Grunberg, N. E. (1990). Variations in food preference and consumption across the menstrual cycle. *Physiol Behav, 47*(2), 287-291.

Bruinsma, K., and Taren, D. L. (1999). Chocolate. Food or drug? *J. Am. Diet. Assoc., 99*, 1249-1256.

Buffenstein, R., Poppitt, S. D., McDevitt, R. M., and Prentice, A. M. (1995). Food intake and the menstrual cycle: a retrospective analysis, with implications for appetite research. *Physiol. Behav., 58*(6), 1067-1077.

Burkman, R., Bell, C., and Serfaty, D. (2011). The evolution of combined oral contraception: improving the risk-to-benefit ratio. *Contraception, 84*(1), 19-34. doi: 10.1016/j.contraception.2010.11.004

Butera, P. C. (2010). Estradiol and the control of food intake. *Physiol. Behav., 99*, 175-180.

Butera, P. C., Bradway, D. M., and Cataldo, N. J. (1993). Modulation of the satiety effect of cholecystokinin by estradiol. *Physiol. Behav., 53*, 1235-1238.

Caro, J. F., Kolaczynski, J. W., Nyce, M. R., Ohannesian, J. P., Opentanova, I., Goldman, W. H., Lynn, R. B., Zhang, P. L., Sinha, M. K., and Considine, R. V. (1996). Decreased cerebrospinal- fluid/serum leptin ratio in obesity: A possible mechanism for leptin resistance. *Lancet, 348*, 159-161.

Channing, C. P., Schaerf, F. W., Anderson, L. D., and Tsafriri, A. (1980). Ovarian follicular and luteal physiology. *Int. Rev. Physiol., 22*, 117-201.

Channon, S., and Hayward, A. (1990). The effect of short-term fasting on processing of food cues in normal subjects. *Int. J. Eat Disord., 9*, 447-452.

Cheikh Ismail, L. I., Al-Hourani, H., Lightowler, H. J., Aldhaheri, A. S., and Henry, C. J. (2009). Energy and nutrient intakes during different phases of the menstrual cycle in females in the United Arab Emirates. *Ann. Nutr. Metab., 54*(2), 124-128.

Chung, S. C., Bond, E. F., and Jarrett, M. E. (2010). Food intake changes across the menstrual cycle in Taiwanese women. *Biol. Res. Nurs., 12*(1), 37-46.

Clegg, D. J., Brown, L. M., Zigman, J. M., Kemp, C. H., Strader, A. D., Benoit, S. C., Woods, S. C., Mangiaracina, M., and Geary, N. (2007). Estradiol-dependent decrease in the orexigenic potency of ghrelin in female rats. *Diabetes, 56*(4), 1051-1058.

Clegg, D. J., Riedy, C. A., Smith, K. A., Benoit, S. C., and Woods, S. C. (2003). Differential sensitivity to central leptin and insulin in male and female rats. *Diabetes, 52*(3), 682-687.

Considine, R. V., Sinha, M. K., Heiman, M. L., Kriauciunas, A., Stephens, T. W., Nyce, M. R., Ohannesian, J. P., Marco, C. C., McKee, L. J., and Bauer, T. L. (1996). Serum immunoreactive-leptin concentrations in normal-weight and obese humans. *N Engl. J. Med., 334*(5), 292-295.

Cotrufo, P., Monteleone, P., d'Istria, M., Fuschino, A., Serino, I., and Maj, M. (2000). Aggressive behavioral characteristics and endogenous hormones in women with Bulimia nervosa. [Clinical Trial]. *Neuropsychobiology, 42*(2), 58-61. doi: 26673

Crave, J., Lejeune, H., Brebant, C., Baret, C., and Pugeat, M. (1995). Differential effects of insulin and insulin-like growth factor I on the production of plasma steroid-binding globulins by human hepatoblastoma derived (Hep G2) cells. *J. Clin. Endocrinol. Metab., 80*, 1283-1289.

Creutz, L. M., and Kritzer, M. F. (2002). Estrogen receptor-beta immunoreactivity in the midbrain of adult rats: regional, subregional, and cellular localization in the A10, A9, and A8 dopamine cell groups. *J. Comp. Neurol., 446*, 288-300.

Cross, G. B., Marley, J., Miles, H., and Willson, K. (2001). Changes in nutrient intake during the menstrual cycle of overweight women with premenstrual syndrome. *Br. J. Nutr., 85*(4), 475-482.

Dafopoulos, K., Sourlas, D., Kallitsaris, A., Pournaras, S., and Messinis, I. E. (2009). Blood ghrelin, resistin, and adiponectin concentrations during the normal menstrual cycle. *Fertil. Steril., 92*, 1389-1394.

Dalvit-McPhillips, S. P. (1983). The effect of the human menstrual cycle on nutrient intake. *Physiol. Behav., 31*(2), 209-212.

Dalvit, S. P. (1981). The effect of the menstrual cycle on patterns of food intake. *Am. J. Clin. Nutr., 34*(9), 1811-1815.

Danker-Hopfe, H., Roczen, K., and Löwenstein-Wagner, U. (1995). Regulation of food intake during the menstrual cycle. *Anthropol Anz, 53*(3), 231-238.

Davidsen, L., Vistisen, B., and Astrup, A. (2007). Impact of the menstrual cycle on determinants of energy balance: a putative role in weight loss attempts. *Int. J. Obes. (Lond), 31*(12), 1777-1785.

Dye, L. (2001). Cravings across the menstrual cycle and in premenstrual syndrome. In M. M. Heatherington (Ed.), *Food Cravings and Addiction* (pp. 365-390). Leatherhead, Surrey, UK: Leatherhead Publishing.

Eck, L. H., Bennett, A. G., Egan, B. M., Ray, J. W., Mitchell, C. O., Smith, M. A., and Klesges, R. C. (1997). Differences in macronutrient selections in users and nonusers of an oral contraceptive. *Am. J. Clin. Nutr., 65*(2), 419-424.

Eckel, L. A. (1999). Ingestive behaviour in female rats: influence of the ovarian cycle. *Appetite, 32*(2), 274.

Flegal, K. M., and Troiano, R. P. (2000). Changes in the distribution of body mass index of adults and children in the US population. *Int. J. Obes. Relat. Metab. Disord., 24*(7), 807-818.

Freeman, M. E. (1988). The ovarian cycle of the rat. In E. Knobil and J. Neil (Eds.), *Physiology of reproduction* (pp. 1893-1928). New York: Raven Press Ltd.

Gallo, M. F., Lopez, L. M., Grimes, D. A., Schulz, K. F., and Helmerhorst, F. M. (2011). Combination contraceptives: effects on weight. *Cochrane Database Syst. Rev.* (9), CD003987.

Gallo, M. F., Nanda, K., Grimes, D. A., Lopez, L. M., and Schulz, K. F. (2008). 20 microg versus >20 microg estrogen combined oral contraceptives for contraception. *Cochrane Database Of Systematic Reviews (Online)*(4), CD003989.

Gambacciani, M., Ciaponi, M., Cappagli, B., Piaggesi, L., De Simone, L., Orlandi, R., and R, G. A. (1997). Body weight, body fat distribution, and hormonal replacement therapy in early postmenopausal women. *J. Clin. Endocrinol. Metab., 82*, 414-417.

Gambineri, A., Repaci, A., Patton, L., Grassi, I., Pocognoli, P., Cognigni, G., Pasqui, F., Pagotto, U., and Pasquali, R. (2009). Prominent role of low HDL-cholesterol in explaining the high prevalence of the metabolic syndrome in polycystic ovary syndrome. *Nutr. Metab. Cardiovasc. Dis., 19*, 797-804.

Gaudet, L. M., Kives, S., Hahn, P. M., and Reid, R. L. (2004). What women believe about oral contraceptives and the effect of counselling. *Contraception, 69*, 31-36.

Geary, N., Asarian, L., Korach, K. S., Pfaff, D. W., and Ogawa, S. (2001). Deficits in E2-dependent control of feeding weight gain, and cholecystokinin satiation in ER-alpha null mice. *Endocrinology, 142*, 4751-4757.

Geiselman, P. J., Martin, J. R., VanderWeele, D. A., and Novin, D. (1981). Dietary self-selection in cycling and neonatally ovariectomized rats. *Appetite, 2*, 87-101.

Gong, E. J., Garrel, D., and Calloway, D. H. (1989). Menstrual cycle and voluntary food intake. *Am. J. Clin. Nutr., 49*(2), 252-258.

Hetherington, M. M., and MacDiarmid, J. I. (1993). "Chocolate addiction": a preliminary study of its description and its relationship to problem eating. *Appetite, 21*(3), 233-246.

Hirschberg, A. L., Bystrom, B., Carlstrom, K., and von Schoultz, B. (1996). Reduced serum cholecystokinin and increase in body fat during oral contraception. *Contraception, 53*(2), 109-113. doi: 0010782495002650 [pii]

Hirschberg, A. L., Naessén, S., Stridsberg, M., Byström, B., and Holte, J. (2004). Impaired cholecystokinin secretion and disturbed appetite regulation in women with polycystic ovary syndrome. *Gynecol. Endocrinol, 19*, 79-87.

Huang, Y. S., Doi, R., Chowdhury, P., Pasley, J. N., Nishikawa, M., Huang, T. J., and Rayford, P. L. (1993). Effect of cholecystokinin on food intake at different stages of the estrous cycle in female rats. *J. Assoc. Acad. Minor. Phys., 4*, 56-58.

Jankowiak, R., and Stern, J. J. (1974). Food intake and body weight modifications following medial hypothalamic hormone implants in female rats. *Physiol. Behav., 12*, 875-881.

Johnson, W. G., Corrigan, S. A., Lemmon, C. R., Bergeron, K. B., and Crusco, A. H. (1994). Energy regulation over the menstrual cycle. *Physiol. Behav.*, *56*(3), 523-527.

Jones, M. E., Thorburn, A. W., Britt, K. L., Hewitt, K. N., Wreford, N. G., Proietto, J., Oz, O. K., Leury, B. J., Robertson, K. M., Yao, S., and Simpson, E. R. (2000). Aromatase-deficient (ArKO) mice have a phenotype of increased adiposity. *PNAS, 7*, 12735-12740.

Karlsson, R., Linden, A., and von Schoultz, B. (1992). Suppression of 24-hour cholecystokinin secretion by oral contraceptives. *Am. J. Obstet. Gynecol.*, *167*(1), 58-59.

Klump, K. L., Keel, P. K., Culbert, K. M., and Edler, C. (2008). Ovarian hormones and binge eating: exploring associations in community samples. *Psychol. Med., 38*, 1749-1757.

Kojima, M., Hosoda, H., Date, Y., Nakazato, M., Matsuo, H., and Kangawa, K. (1999). Ghrelin is a growth-hormone-releasing acylated peptide from stomach. *Nature, 402*, 656-660.

Lara-Torre, E. (2009). Update in adolescent contraception. *Obstet. Gynecol. Clin. North Am., 36*, 119-128.

Le Saux, M., Morissette, M., and Di Paolo, T. (2006). ER[beta] mediates the estradiol increase of D2 receptors in rat striatum and nucleus accumbens. *Neuropharmacology, 50*, 451-457.

Le, Y. C., Rahman, M., and Berenson, A. B. (2009). Early weight gain predicting later weight gain among depot medroxyprogesterone acetate users. *Obstet. Gynecol., 114*(2 Pt 1), 279-284.

Leibowitz, S. F., Akabayashi, A., Alexander, J. T., and Wang, J. (1998). Gonadal steriods and hypothalamic galanin and neuropeptide Y:role in eating behavior and body weight control in female rats. *Endocrinology, 139*(4), 1771-1780.

Leiman, G. (1972). Depo-medroxyprogesterone acetate as a contraceptive agent: its effect on weight and blood pressure. *Am. J. Obstet. Gynecol., 114*(1), 97-102.

Li, E. T., Tsang, L. B., and Lui, S. S. (1999). Menstrual cycle and voluntary food intake in young Chinese women. *Appetite, 33*(1), 109-118.

Liang, Y. Q., Akishita, M., Kim, S., Ako, J., Hashimoto, M., Iijima, K., Ohike, Y., Watanabe, T., Sudoh, N., Toba, K., Yoshizumi, M., and Ouchi, Y. (2002). Estrogen receptor beta is involved in the anorectic action of estrogen. *Int. J. Obes. Relat. Metab. Disord, 26*(8), 1103-1109.

Lindh, I., Blohm, F., Andersson-Ellström, A., and Milsom, I. (2009). Contraceptive use and pregnancy outcome in three generations of Swedish female teenagers from the same urban population. *Contraception, 80*(2), 163-169.

Lindh, I., Ellström, A. A., and Milsom, I. (2011). The long-term influence of combined oral contraceptives on body weight. *Hum. Reprod., 26*(7), 1917-1924.

Lyons, P. M., Truswell, A. S., Mira, M., Vizzard, J., and Abraham, S. F. (1989). Reduction of food intake in the ovulatory phase of the menstrual cycle. *Am. J. Clin. Nutr., 49*(6), 1164-1168.

Maltoni, M., Nanni, O., Scarpi, E., Rossi, D., Serra, P., and Amadori, D. (2001). High-dose progestins for the treatment of cancer anorexia-cachexia syndrome: a systematic review of randomised clinical trials. *Ann. Oncol., 12*, 289-300.

Martini, M. C., Lampe, J. W., Slavin, J. L., and Kurzer, M. S. (1994). Effect of the menstrual cycle on energy and nutrient intake. *Am. J. Clin. Nutr., 60*(6), 895-899.

Massé, P. G. (1991). Nutrient intakes of women who use oral contraceptives. *J. Am. Diet Assoc., 91*(9), 1118-1120.

McNeill, G., Bruce, A. C., Ross, E., and James, W. P. T. (1988). Energy balance in women using oral contraceptives. *Proc Nutr Soc, 47*(58A).

Michalakis, K., Mintziori, G., Kaprara, A., Tarlatzis, B. C., and Goulis, D. G. (2012). The complex interaction between obesity, metabolic syndrome and reproductive axis: A narrative review. *Metabolism, Epub ahead of print.*

Michener, W., Rozin, P., Freeman, E., and Gale, L. (1999). The role of low progesterone and tension as triggers of perimenstrual chocolate and sweets craving: some negative experimental evidence. *Physiol. Behav., 67*(3), 417-420.

Mishell, D. R. (2004). State of the art in hormonal contraception: An overview. *Am. J. Obstet. Gynecol., 190*(4), S1-S4.

Mogri, M., Dhindsa, S., Quattrin, T., Ghanim, H., and Dandona, P. (2012). Testosterone Concentrations In Young Pubertal And Post-Pubertal Obese Males. *Clin. Endocrinol. (Oxf), Epub ahead of print.*

Morton, G. J., and Schwartz, M. W. (2001). The NPY/AgRP neuron and energy homeostasis. *Int. J. Obes., 25*(5), S56–S62.

Musatov, S., Chen, W., Pfaff, D. W., Mobbs, C. V., Yang, X. J., Clegg, D. J., Kaplitt, M. G., and Ogawa, S. (2007). Silencing of estrogen receptor alpha in the ventromedial nucleus of hypothalamus leads to metabolic syndrome. *Proc. Natl. Acad. Sci. USA, 104*(7), 2501-2506.

Naessén, S., Carlström, K., Byström, B., Pierre, Y., and Hirschberg, A. L. (2007). Effects of an antiandrogenic oral contraceptive on appetite and eating behavior in bulimic women. *Psychoneuroendocrinology, 32*(5), 548-554.

Oddens, B. J. (1999). Women's satisfaction with birth control: a population survey of physical and psychological effects of oral contraceptives, intrauterine devices, condoms, natural family planning, and sterilization among 1466 women. *Contraception, 59*(5), 277-286.

Olofsson, L. E., Pierce, A. A., and Xu, A. W. (2009). Functional requirement of AgRP and NPY neurons in ovarian cycle-dependent regulation of food intake. *Proc. Natl. Acad. Sci. USA, 106*(37), 15932-15937.

Owen, J. A. J. (1975). Physiology of the menstrual cycle. *Am. J. Clin. Nutr., 28*, 333-338.

Pelchat, M. L. (1997). Food cravings in young and elderly adults. *Appetite, 28*, 103-113.

Pelkman, C. L., Heinbach, R. A., and Rolls, B. J. (2000). Reproductive hormones and eating behavior in young women. *Appetite, 34*(2), 217-218.

Pelleymounter, M. A., Baker, M. B., and McCaleb, M. (1999). Does estradiol mediate leptin's effects on adiposity and body weight? *Am. J. Physiol., 276*, E955-E963.

Pliner, P., and Fleming, A. S. (1983). Food intake, body weight, and sweetness preferences over the menstrual cycle in humans. *Physiol. Behav., 30*(4), 663-666.

Pohle-Krauza, R. J., Carey, K. H., and Pelkman, C. L. (2008). Dietary restraint and menstrual cycle phase modulated L-phenylalanine-induced satiety. *Physiol. Behav., 93*(4-5), 851-861.

Poretsky, L. (1991). On the paradox of insulin-induced hyperandrogenism in insulin-resistant states. *Endocr. Rev., 12*, 3-13.

Price, T. M., O'Brien, S. N., Welter, B. H., George, R., Anandjiwala, J., and Kilgore, M. (1998). Estrogen regulation of adipose tissue lipoprotein lipase-possible mechanism of body fat distribution. *Am. J. Obstet. Gynecol., 178*, 101-107.

Procter-Gray, E., Cobb, K. L., Crawford, S. L., Bachrach, L. K., Chirra, A., Sowers, M., Greendale, G. A., Nieves, J. W., Kent, K., and Kelsey, J. L. (2008). Effect of oral contraceptives on weight and body composition in young female runners. *Med. Sci. Sports Exerc., 40*(7), 1205-1212.

Quarta, C., Mazza, R., Pasquali, R., and Pagotto, U. (2012). Role of sex hormones in modulation of brown adipose tissue activity. *J. Mol. Endocrinol., 49*(1), R1-7.

Rapkin, A. J., Edelmuth, E., Chang, L. C., Reading, A. E., McGuire, M. T., and Su, T. P. (1987). Whole blood serotonin in premenstrual syndrome. *Obstet. Gynecol., 70*, 533-537.

Richard, D. (1986). Effects of ovarian hormones on energy balance and brown adipose tissue thermogenesis. *Am. J. Physiol., 250*, R245-249.

Risser, W. L., Gefter, L. R., Barratt, M. S., and Risser, J. M. (1999). Weight change in adolescents who used hormonal contraception. *J. Adolesc. Health, 24*, 433-436.

Rodin, J., Mancuso, J., Granger, J., and Nelbach, E. (1991). Food cravings in relation to body mass index, restraint and estradiol levels. A repeated measures study in healthy women. *Appetite, 17*, 177-185.

Roesch, D. M. (2006). Effects of selective estrogen receptor agonists on food intake and body weight gain in rats. *Physiol. Behav., 87*, 39-44.

Rosenberg, M. J., and Waugh, M. S. (1998). Oral contraceptive discontinuation: a prospective evaluation of frequency and reasons. *Am. J. Obstet. Gynecol., 179*, 577-582.

Shughrue, P. J., Lane, M. V., and Merchenthaler, I. (1997). Comparative distribution of estrogen receptor-alpha and -beta mRNA in the rat central nervous system. *J. Comp. Neurol., 388*, 507-525.

Sitruk-Ware, R. (2006). New progestagens for contraceptive use. *Hum. Reprod. Update, 12*(2), 169-178.

Smith, G. P., and Gibbs, J. (1992). The development and proof of the CCK hypothesis of satiety. In C. T. Dourish, S. J. Cooper, S. D. Iversen and L. L. Ivesen (Eds.), *Multiple cholecystokinin receptors in the CNS* (pp. 166-182). Oxford: Oxford Univ Press.

Sundblad, C., Landen, M., Eriksson, T., Bergman, L., and Eriksson, E. (2005). Effects of the androgen antagonist flutamide and the serotonin reuptake inhibitor citalopram in bulimia nervosa: a placebo-controlled pilot study. *J. Clin. Psychopharmacol., 25*(1), 85-88.

Titolo, D., Cai, F., and Belsham, D. D. (2006). Coordinate regulation of neuropeptide Y and agouti-related peptide gene expression by estrogen depends on the ratio of estrogen receptor (ER) alpha to ERbeta in clonal hypothalamic neurons. *Mol. Endocrinol., 20*(9), 2080-2092.

Tucci, S. A., Murphy, L. E., Boyland, E. J., Dye, L., and Halford, J. C. (2010). Oral contraceptive effects on food choice during the follicular and luteal phases of the menstrual cycle. A laboratory based study. *Appetite, 55*(3), 388-392.

Tucci, S. A., Murphy, L. E., Boyland, E. J., and Halford, J. C. (2009). Influence of premenstrual syndrome and oral contraceptive effects on food choice during the follicular and luteal phase of the menstrual cycle. *Endocrinol. Nutr., 56*(4), 170-175.

Tucci, S. A., Parkes, R., McCann, L., Boyland, E. J., Harrold, J. A., and Halford, J. C. G. (2011). *Effects of oral contraceptives on intake of snack food items.* Paper presented at the 18th European Congress on Obesity, Istanbul, Turkey.

United Nations, Department of Economic and Social Affairs, Population Division. World contraceptive use (2011), from http://www.un.org/esa/population/publications/contraceptive2011/contraceptive2011.htm

Wade, G. N. (1975). Some effects of ovarian hormones on food intake and body weight in female rats. *J. Comp. Physiol. Psychol., 88*, 183-193.

Wade, G. N., and Schneider, J. E. (1992). Metabolic fuels and reproduction in female mammals. *Neurosci. Biobehav. Rev., 16*, 235-272.

Wallace, R. B., Heiss, G., Burrows, B., and Graves, K. (1987). Contrasting diet and body mass among users and nonusers of oral contraceptives and exogenous estrogens: the Lipid Research Clinics Program Prevalence Study. *Am. J. Epidemiol., 125*(5), 854-859.

Wanyonyi, S. Z., Stones, W. R., and Sequeira, E. (2011). Health-related quality of life changes among users of depot medroxyprogesterone acetate for contraception. *Contraception, 84*(5), e17-e22.

Warholm, L., Petersen, K. R., and Ravn, P. (2012). Combined oral contraceptives' influence on weight, body composition, height, and bone mineral density in girls younger than 18 years: A systematic review. *Eur. J. Contracept Reprod. Health Care, 17*(4), 245-253.

Weingarten, H. P., and Elston, D. (1991). Food cravings in a college population. *Appetite, 17*, 167-175.

Westhoff, C. L., Heartwell, S., Edwards, S., Zieman, M., Stuart, G., Cwiak, C., Davis, A., Robilotto, T., Cushman, L., and Kalmuss, D. (2007). Oral contraceptive discontinuation: do side effects matter? *Am. J. Obstet. Gynecol., 196*(4), 412 e411-e417.

Wysocki, S. (2000). A survey of American women regarding the use of oral contraceptives and weight gain. *Int J Gynecol Obstet, 70*(Suppl. 1), 114.

Yonkers, K. A., O'Brien, P. M. S., and Eriksson, E. (2008). Premenstrual syndrome. *Lancet, 371*, 1200-1210.

Zellner, D. A., Garriga-Trillo, A., Centeno, S., and Wadsworth, E. (2004). Chocolate craving and the menstrual cycle. *Appetite, 42*(1), 119-121.

Zellner, D. A., Garriga-Trillo, A., Rohm, E., Centeno, S., and Parker, S. (1999). Food liking and craving: a cross-cultural approach. *Appetite, 33*, 61-70.

ISBN: 978-1-62417-945-7
© 2013 Nova Science Publishers, Inc.

Chapter V

No Changes in Energy Intake, Resting and Physical Activity Energy Expenditure, or Food Reinforcement Across the Menstrual Cycle

Jessica McNeil, Jameason D. Cameron and Éric Doucet[*]
Behavioural and Metabolic Research Unit,
School of Human Kinetics
University of Ottawa. Ottawa, Ontario, Canada

Abstract

Background: Energy intake (EI) and physical activity energy expenditure (PAEE) have been previously evaluated across the menstrual cycle with food and physical activity journals. To our knowledge, the direct assessments of EI, macronutrient intake, resting energy expenditureEE (REE) and PAEE have not been studied across the

[*] Send correspondence and reprint requests to: Éric Doucet, Ph.D. Behavioural and Metabolic Research Unit (BMRU) School of Human Kinetics University of Ottawa Ottawa (On), Canada, K1N 6N5 Phone: 1-613-562-5800 ext.: 7364 Fax: 1-613-562-5291 E-mail: edoucet@uottawa.ca

menstrual cycle within the same study design. Furthermore, no study has related these factors to possible variations in the severity of the premenstrual syndrome (PMS) and food reinforcement across the cycle.

Methods: Seventeen women (Body mass index: 22.3 ± 1.6 kg/m²; Body fat-DXA: $28.5\pm6.8\%$) participated in three identical sessions during distinct phases of the menstrual cycle: Early follicular, Late follicular/ovulation and Mid-luteal (confirmed by basal temperature and plasma gonadotropins, estradiol and progesterone levels). EI was measured inside the laboratory and under free-living conditions with food menus and food journals, respectively. REE and PAEE were measured with indirect calorimetry and accelerometers, respectively. Also measured were body fat mass (DXA), the severity of PMS, leptin and the relative- reinforcing value (RRV) of preferred foods.

Results: No differences in body fat mass, REE, PAEE and leptin were noted across the menstrual cycle. Furthermore, no changes in measured and reported energy, carbohydrate, lipid and protein intakes, as well as the RRV of preferred foods were noted across the cycle. Differences in the severity of PMS (25 ± 10, 19 ± 11, 25 ± 10 points; $p<0.05$) across phases were noted. However, the severity of PMS and food reinforcement did not coincide with energy and macronutrient intakes.

Conclusions: Taken together, these results suggest that the menstrual cycle may not be of practical concern when assessing food intake and physical activity patterns under the methodological conditions presented in this study.

Keywords: menstrual cycle, energy intake, resting energy expenditure, physical activity energy expenditure, food reinforcement, premenstrual syndrome

Introduction

It has been previously observed that energy intake (EI) decreases during the late follicular and ovulation phases of the menstrual cycle, which are characterized by higher levels of estradiol, while EI tends to increase during the luteal phase, at which time levels of both estradiol and progesterone are elevated [1]. A large variation can however be observed when comparing the caloric intake values previously reported, with increases in EI ranging from ≈364-2092 kilojoules (kj) during the luteal phase in comparison to the follicular phase. As for macronutrient intake across the menstrual cycle, most studies [2-7] noted similar results: increases in absolute intake of all macronutrients during the luteal phase.

As for resting energy expenditure (REE), a mean increase in basal metabolic rate of 15% following ovulation has been previously noted [8]. However, not all participants haddemonstrated an increase in basal metabolic rate following ovulation [8].

As for physical activity energy expenditure (PAEE), no variation has been noted across the menstrual cycle with physical activity journals [2]. Lastly, no significant changes in body weight or body fat percentage across the cycle have been previously noted in lean women [2; 3; 9].

Certain secondary factors may in part explain the possible variations in EI, REE and PAEE across the menstrual cycle. Among those are the occurrence and severity of the premenstrual syndrome (PMS). Approximately 50% of women suffer from a minimal level of distress related to PMS, from which 31%, 14% and 8% reported low, moderate and severe levels of distress, respectively [10]. Women who also reported more severe PMS symptoms consumed on average more calories, and had more frequent episodes of overeating and cravings for sweet-fatty foods during the late luteal phase [11; 12]. Additionally, the relative-reinforcing value (RRV) of food, a specific aspect of appetitive motivation which can be generally portrayed as the amount of work/effort one individual is willing to do in order to obtain a certain type of food [13], has not been previously evaluated across the menstrual cycle. The RRV of food is an objective measure that may in part explain the possible variations in energy and snack intake across the cycle, especially at times during which women may be more prone to episodes of overeating [14]. Finally, variations in leptin levels, a hormone that is secreted by adipocytes and circulates in the plasma at concentrations relative to fat mass [15], have been noted across the menstrual cycle; with values ≈35-60% higher during the early to mid-luteal phase in comparison to the early follicular phase [9; 16-19].

The objective of this study was to measure EI, macronutrient intake, REE and PAEE across the menstrual cycle within the same study design. In an effort to increase the accuracy of menstrual cycle phase determination, plasma levels of LH, FSH, estradiol and progesterone, as well as basal temperature were assessed at the start of every experimental session. We hypothesized that energy, carbohydrate, lipid and preferred snack intakes would be highest during the mid-luteal phase; coinciding with more severe PMS symptoms and greater reinforcement for snack foods. We also hypothesized that leptin levels would be higher during the mid-luteal phase. Lastly, we hypothesized that no changes in body weight, body fat percentage, REE and PAEE would occur across the cycle.

Materials and Methods

Participants

A total of 18 women completed this study. However, one participant was excluded from the analysis due to her measured LH, estradiol and progesterone levels being well below the normal range [20], suggesting that an anovulatory cycle may have occurred.

And so, the results of 17 participants are presented herein. Participants had to be between the ages of 18-40 years, non-smokers, weight stable (± 2 kg), have a 24-34 day menstrual cycle, not taking prescribed medications, and not taking hormonal contraceptives (e.g. pill, patch, injection, intra-uterine device) within the past six months. This study was conducted according to the guidelines laid down in the Declaration of Helsinki and all the procedures involving human participants were approved by the University of Ottawa ethics committee. Written informed consent was also obtained from all participants.

Design and Procedure

A preliminary session was held to determine whether participants corresponded to the inclusion criteria. Following this, three identical experimental sessions were conducted during the early follicular (days 1-5 inclusively), late follicular/ovulation (days 11-14 inclusively) and mid-luteal (days 21-26 inclusively) phases.

These days were based on a 28-day cycle and each participant was asked to count the number of days (length) of her menstrual cycle for at least one month prior to testing; permitting us to tailor the times of testing for each participant according to the length of her cycle. Plasma LH, FSH, estradiol and progesterone levels, as well as basal temperature, aided in confirming each menstrual cycle phase. Lastly, the participants arrived at the laboratory at 8h00 following a 12-hour overnight fast prior to the start of each experimental session.

Participants had also been instructed to not consume any alcohol or engage in any type of structured physical activity (e.g. playing sports or training) for at least 24 hours prior to the start of each session. Anthropometric measurements were performed during the preliminary and each experimental session, while all other measurements described below were performed during the three experimental sessions.

Anthropometric Measurements

Standing height was measured, without shoes, to the nearest centimeter using a Tanita HR-100 height rod (Tanita Corporation of America, Inc, Arlington Heights, IL). Body weight and body composition were measured using a standard beam scale (HR-100; BWB-800AS, Tanita Corporation, Arlington Heights, IL., USA) and DXA scanner (Lunar Prodigy, General Electric, Madison, WI, USA), respectively. During each experimental session, anthropometric measurements were taken at 9h00. The coefficient of variation and correlation for body fat percentage measured by DXA scanner in 12 healthy participants were 1.8% and $r = 0.99$, respectively.

Blood Sample

A single blood sample was drawn from the antecubital vein of the non-dominant arm between 9h00 and 9h30 to determine the plasma levels of estradiol, progesterone, FSH, LH and leptin. Each blood sample was placed into a tube containing ethylenediaminetetraacetic acid (EDTA) and was centrifuged at 3500 rpm at 4^0C immediately after the blood was drawn and stored at -80^0C until assayed. LH and FSH levels were assayed with a two step "sandwich" chemiluminescent assay (CIA) using the Beckman Coulter Dxl Unicel 800 (Beckman Coulter Canada Incorporated, Mississauga, Ontario, Canada).

Progesterone levels were assayed by means of an electro-chemiluminescent immunoassay (ECLIA) system, Elecsys 2010 disk system (Roche Diagnostics, Indianapolis, Indiana, USA). As for estradiol analyses, a carbonyl metallo immunoassay (CMIA) procedure was employed with an Architect estradiol reagent kit (Abbott Laboratories, Abbott Park, Illinois, USA). 100 test reagent packs were used to analyze gonadotropins, estradiol and progesterone levels. Leptin levels were assayed with a dual range enzyme-linked immunosorbent assay (ELISA) human leptin kit (Millipore Corporation, Billerica, Massachusetts, USA). Leptin concentrations were determined as the average of duplicate determinations and the duplicate coefficient of variation was 7.4%.

Temperature Measurements

Basal temperature was measured orally with a digital thermometer (rapid digital thermometer, BD, Franklin Lakes, NJ, USA) between 9h00 and 9h30.

Energy Intake

EI and the macronutrient composition of foods during each laboratory session were evaluated with a validated food menu [21]. This food menu contains 62 items, which includes breakfast items, snacks, hot meals, caloric beverages and water. The participants were handed a copy of the food menu on six different occasions throughout the day (9h30, 10h30, 12h30, 14h30, 15h30 and 16h30), at which time they were able to choose the type of foods and beverages from the menu that they may want to consume. The chosen foods and beverages were then prepared and served to the participants in a sufficient amount (two portions of each item). The prepared foods were weighed in grams before serving, using an electronic scale (Scout Pro SP2001, Ohaus Corporation, Pine Brook, N.J.), and after the participants were done eating. The macronutrient composition of foods consumed were analyzed with nutritional labels and the Food Processor SQL software (version 9.6.2; ESHA Research, Salem, OR). At the end of each experimental session, a weighed food journal [22] was given to the participants to record food and beverage intakes outside of the laboratory for three consecutive days following each session. Participants were asked to report, as accurately as possible, the foods and beverages consumed (i.e. brand name and type of food/recipe), the location and time at which they were consumed, and the quantities for each, estimated using standard household items (e.g. cups, tablespoons). Finally, participants were asked to provide, if possible, recipes and/or dietary information for all items consumed.

Pleasantness Ratings of Foods and Beverages Consumed

Participants were asked to draw a vertical line on a 150 millimeter visual analogue scale (VAS) [23], reflecting their appreciation for all foods consumed during each experimental session. The question asked on each VAS was: "How pleasant is the taste of this food?" The pleasantness rating of each item was performed in order to determine whether participants enjoyed/liked the foods and beverages consumed, and evaluate whether this may alter with menstrual cycle phase.

Energy Expenditure

REE was measured using indirect calorimetry (Vmax encore 29N, Viasys respiratory care Incorporated, Palm Springs, California, USA) at 8h30, for 30 minutes. The participants rested in a supine position for 30 minutes prior to the start of REE measurement. The coefficient of variation and correlation for the REE measured by the Vmax encore 29N system in 12 healthy participants were 5.1% and $r = 0.94$, respectively. As for PAEE, this was estimated with a small, water resistant, omnidirectional accelerometer (Actical Accelerometer, Bio-Lynx Scientific Equipment, Montreal, Quebec, Canada) for seven consecutive days following each session. Participants were asked to wear the accelerometer at all times (including in water), from the time they wake until the time they went to sleep. The accelerometer was worn on the right hip (anterior to the iliac crest), and secured with an elastic belt with the arrow pointing up, because that placement, when evaluated along with lower leg or foot, upper leg, head and trunk, lower arm or hand, and upper arm placements, was the best predictor of energy expenditure ($r = 0.92 - 0.97$) [24]. The accelerometers used in this study were previously validated with doubly labelled water measurements [25].

Shortened Premenstrual Assessment Form

The occurrence and severity of PMS was evaluated with the shortened premenstrual assessment form [26] at 9h30. This questionnaire is used to classify the subjective changes in certain mood and physical symptoms (i.e. affect, water retention and pain), based on a six-point visual analogue scale (1 = no change and 6 = extreme change), seen or felt by the participants at the time of measurement using a ten category (symptom) chart.

Relative-Reinforcing Value of Food

The RRV of a preferred snack food versus a preferred vegetable or fruit was measured with the Behavioral Choice Task [13] using progressive ratios for responding, as previously described [27]. A small sample of each participant's favorite snack and favorite fruit/vegetable was presented to them prior to the test at 11h30. and tThey were then asked to consume both samples. Following this, the participants earned points by working for the two personalized food items of choice. The participants then received a specific amount of each food item at 13h00 based on their point distribution during the test; a ratio of 1 slice/piece ($\approx$ 4-5 grams) of the preferred food was given for each point earned towards that food reinforcer. Preferred snack and vegetable/fruit intakes were also measured.

Statistical Analyses

Statistical analyses were performed using SPSS software (version 17.0; SPSS Inc, Chicago, IL). A two-way repeated measures ANOVA was used to determine the main effects of menstrual cycle phase (early follicular, late follicular/ovulation and mid-luteal) on the components of dietary intake (total amount of energy (kJ), protein (kJ), carbohydrate (kJ) and lipid (kJ)) for the in-laboratory sessions and the three-day weighed food journals, hormone levels (FSH, LH, estradiol, progesterone and leptin), REE, PAEE, reported PMS, as well as the RRV of snack and fruit/vegetable and the associated consumption of each preferred food. ANOVA Bonferroni tests were used to evaluate where significant differences existed. Bivariate correlations were used to determine the strength of the relationship between measured and reported energy and macronutrient intakes with reported PMS and the RRV of food points, button presses and the consumption of preferred snacks and fruits/vegetables. Values are presented as means $\pm$ standard deviations. Differences with p-values < 0.05 were considered statistically significant.

Results

Characteristics of the Participants

The characteristics of the participants are shown in Table 1. The average age, height and cycle length of the participants were 22.4±3.2 years, 164.2±0.06 centimeters and 28.1±3.8 days, respectively. There were no significant differences in body weight, body mass index, body fat percentage and fat mass across the menstrual cycle. However, a significant difference was noted in fat-free mass across the menstrual cycle, where fat-free mass was higher during the early follicular phase in comparison to the late follicular/ovulation phase (p<0.05).

Table 1. Characteristics of the participants measured during each menstrual cycle phase for one complete menstrual cycle

	Early Follicular		Late Follicular/ Ovulation		Mid-Luteal		
	Mean	SD	Mean	SD	Mean	SD	Phase (p-value)
Body weight (kg)	60.5	7.5	60.3	7.4	60.4	7.4	NS
BMI (kg/m²)	22.4	1.8	22.3	1.6	22.3	1.6	NS
Fat mass (%)	28.0	6.7	28.3	6.9	28.2	6.9	NS
Fat mass (kg)	17.1	5.9	17.3	6.1	17.3	6.1	NS
Fat-free mass (kg)	42.9	3.2	42.5	3.3	42.7	3.2	0.019

Note: BMI, body mass index; SD, standard deviation; kg, kilogram; m, meter.

Hormone Levels and Basal Temperature

No significant difference was noted in basal temperature across the menstrual cycle (36.1±0.4°C, 36.2±0.4°C, 36.2±0.4°C; p=NS). However, significant differences were noted for FSH (5±2, 6±2, 4±2 IU/L; p<0.0001), LH (4±3, 9±7, 6±6 IU/L; p<0.05), estradiol (93±74, 284±294, 445±154 pmol/L; p<0.005) and progesterone (2.7±1.0, 2.4±1.0, 37.6±25.2 nmol/L; p<0.0001) levels.

As expected, FSH and LH levels were higher during the late follicular/ovulation phase, in comparison to the mid-luteal (p<0.0001) and early follicular (p<0.05) phases. Estradiol levels were higher during the mid-luteal phase than the early follicular phase (p<0.0001).

Progesterone levels were also highest during the mid-luteal phase, when compared to the early follicular (p<0.0001) and late follicular/ovulation (p<0.0001) phases. No significant differences in leptin concentrations (12.2±10.1, 11.3±11.1, 11.5±11.0 ng/ml; p=NS) across the menstrual cycle were noted.

EI, Macronutrient Intake, REE, PAEE and Pleasantness Ratings

As shown in Figure 1, no significant differences were noted for measured (in-laboratory) energy, carbohydrate, lipid and protein intakes across the menstrual cycle. No significant differences in total reported (three-day weighed food journal) energy, carbohydrate, lipid and protein intakes were also noted across the cycle (Figure 2). Additionally, Figure 3 demonstrates that there were no significant differences in REE and PAEE across the menstrual cycle. Lastly, no significant difference in the pleasantness ratings of foods and beverages consumed were noted between menstrual cycle phase (122±17; 124±14, 120±16 mm; p=NS).

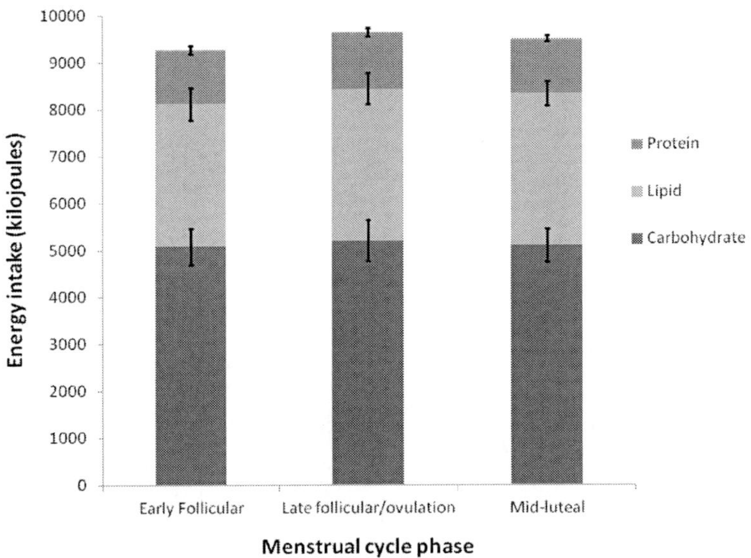

Figure 1. Measured (In-lab from 9h30 to 17h30) energy and macronutrient intakes across the menstrual cycle. Values are presented as means for 17 women with standard errors of the mean represented by vertical bars.

The Occurrence and Severity of PMS and the RRV of Food

A significant difference in the severity of PMS symptoms was noted across the menstrual cycle (25±10, 19±11, 25±10 points; p<0.05). More specifically, a significant difference in the severity of PMS was noted between the late follicular/ovulation and mid-luteal phases (p<0.05).

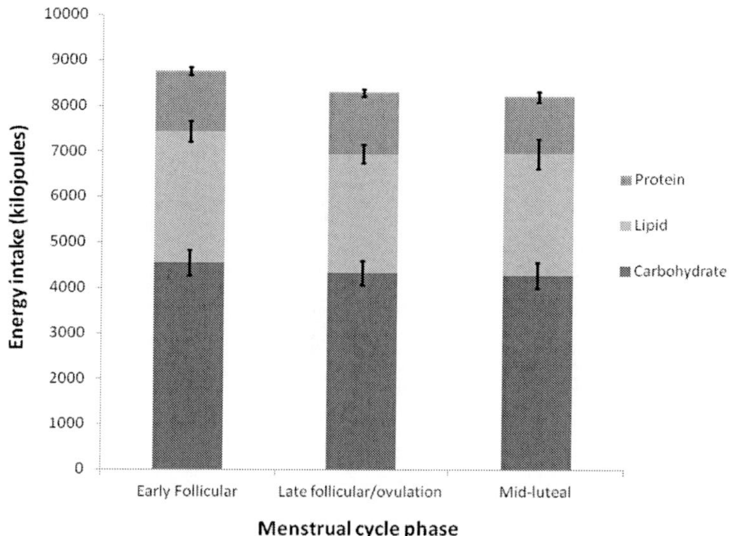

Figure 2. Reported (three-day weighed food journal) energy and macronutrient intakes across the menstrual cycle. Values are presented as means for 17 women with standard errors of the mean represented by vertical bars.

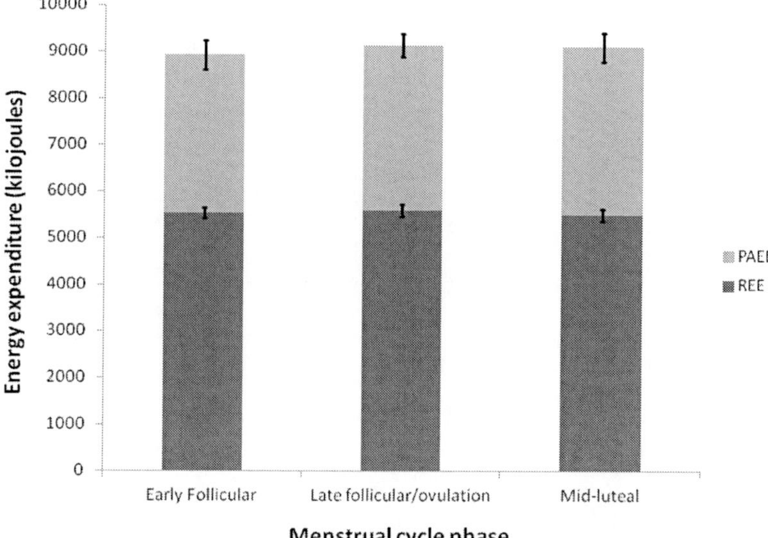

Figure 3. Resting energy expenditure (REE) (measured for 30 minutes) and daily physical activity energy expenditure (PAEE) (measured for seven days) across the menstrual cycle. Values are presented as means for 17 women with standard errors of the mean represented by vertical bars.

However, no correlations were noted between reported and measured energy and macronutrient intakes with the severity of PMS. As for food reinforcement, no significant differences were found in snack points, fruit/vegetable points, snack button presses, fruit/vegetable button presses and percentage of snack points earned across the menstrual cycle (Table 2)

No correlations were found between reported and measured energy and macronutrient intakes with all variables of RRV of food and preferred food intakes. A trend was noted for preferred snack intake across the menstrual cycle (Table 2). However, no significant difference was noted in preferred fruit/vegetable intake across the cycle. Positive correlations were noted between preferred fruit intake and fruit points during the early follicular ($r=0.510$, $p<0.05$), late follicular/ovulation ($r=0.647$, $p<0.01$) and mid-luteal ($r=0.730$, $p<0.01$) phases, as well as between preferred fruit intake and fruit button presses during the late follicular/ovulation ($r=0.620$, $p<0.01$) and mid-luteal ($r=0.688$, $p<0.01$) phases. Positive correlations were also noted between preferred snack intake and snack points ($r=0.510$, $p<0.05$), as well as snack button presses ($r=0.534$, $p<0.05$), but only during the early follicular phase. Lastly, no significant correlations were noted between all variables of RRV of food and the severity of PMS for all tested phases of the menstrual cycle (results not shown).

Table 2. Relative-reinforcing value of food computer task results and preferred snack and fruit/vegetable intakes measured during each menstrual cycle phase for one complete menstrual cycle

	Early Follicular		Late Follicular /Ovulation		Mid-Luteal		
	Mean	SD	Mean	SD	Mean	SD	Phase (p-value)
Snack points	8	5	9	5	10	5	NS
Fruit/vegetable points	12	5	11	5	10	5	NS
Snack button presses	89	68	111	74	126	61	NS
Fruit/vegetable button presses	77	31	67	34	60	28	NS
% snack points	39.4	26.7	46.2	27.2	52.4	22.6	NS
Snack intake (kJ)	431	515	414	347	699	598	0.06
Fruit/vegetable intake (kJ)	247	213	218	121	243	163	NS

Note: SD, standard deviation; kJ, kilojoule.

Discussion

Our results show no differences in measured and reported energy, carbohydrate, lipid and protein intakes across the menstrual cycle, while only a trend was observed in preferred snack intake across the cycle. Additionally, the severity of PMS and food reinforcement were not related to energy and macronutrient intakes. As for preferred snack intake, this was only positively correlated with snack points and snack button presses during the early follicular phase. Thus, our results do not support our initial hypothesis. Leptin did not increase during the mid-luteal phase, which also rejects one of our hypotheses. Lastly, no changes in body weight, body fat percentage, REE and PAEE were noted across the menstrual cycle, thereby accepting our final hypothesis.

No significant variations were noted in basal temperature across the menstrual cycle. However, greater levels of FSH and LH during the late follicular/ovulation phase, as well as higher levels of progesterone during the mid-luteal phase are suggestive that ovulation did occur.

As for anthropometric measurements, no variations in body weight, body mass index, body fat percentage and fat mass were seen across the menstrual cycle, which is in accordance with existing literature [2; 3; 9]. However, a significant difference in fat-free mass was noted between the early follicular and late follicular/ovulation phases. This difference may be due to increases in water retention during the early follicular phase [28], since drops in progesterone levels prior to the start of menses have shown to increase water and salt retention [29] at this time [29].

No significant differences were noted in energy and macronutrient intakes across the menstrual cycle when directly assessed inside the laboratory, as well as reported with three-day weighed food journals. Many studies which have previously evaluated variations in energy and macronutrient intakes across the menstrual cycle have noted significantly higher EI [2-7; 30-32], lipid [2; 3; 5; 7] and carbohydrate [3; 6] intakes during the luteal phase. However, the use of different methodologies and testing times and/or frequencies to assess EI may explain the divergence in the results obtained by these studies. A few studies [3; 6; 7] which noted higher variations in EI have employed dietary recall methods or food journals, and have measured this variable on two occasions (follicular and luteal phases). On the other hand, studies which have directly measured EI inside the laboratory for more than one meal found smaller variations in the latter across the cycle [32; 33]. For instance, Lissner *et al.*

[32] noted an increase of 364 kJ in the luteal phase when compared to the follicular phase. Fong and Kretsch [33] also directly measured *ad libitum* energy and macronutrient intakes inside the laboratory during four phases of the menstrual cycle (menses, follicular, ovulation and luteal) in nine lean women. They noted a trend in carbohydrate intake but no significant difference in EI across the menstrual cycle, which is in accordance with our results. The pleasantness ratings of foods consumed were relatively high (81, 83 and 80% rating on VAS) and showed no significant variations across the menstrual cycle, suggesting that the foods consumed inside the laboratory were overall well appreciated during each session. As for measurements of REE, no significant differences were noted across the menstrual cycle. The highest REE values in this study were noted during the late follicular/ovulation phase, but this was not significant. As for daily PAEE, this study extends results from a previous study that measured PAEE with questionnaires [2], by providing objective measures of PAEE with accelerometers.

Even though many studies [9; 16-19] have noted significant variations in leptin levels across the menstrual cycle, other studies [34-36] have noted no variation in this hormone across the cycle, which is in agreement with our results. The discrepancy between these studies may be in part related to the frequency at which measurements of leptin were taken. The studies which measured leptin levels on four or more occasions across the cycle reported significant variations of this hormone [9; 16-19]. Some of these studies [9; 16-18] even measured leptin from blood samples taken every two-three days for one entire menstrual cycle. On the other hand, the present study and others [34-36] which noted no variation in leptin only assayed blood samples for leptin on three occasions across the cycle, thus suggesting that frequent measurements of leptin may be needed to pick-up significant variations in this hormone across the menstrual cycle.

Reported PMS symptoms were less severe during the late follicular/ovulation phase, which is in accordance with other studies [11; 12; 37]. Despite reporting more severe PMS symptoms during the mid-luteal phase, EI was not higher during this phase. Along those lines, Bryant *et al.* [38] found no significant differences in EI during the follicular and luteal phases in women who reported suffering from PMS, when compared to women who reported not suffering from PMS. Additionally, although not significant, the women who reported suffering from PMS consumed more calories during the follicular phase, which is similar to the findings of the current study even though PMS symptoms were not greater at this time.

The present study is one of the first to measure the RRV of preferred foods across the menstrual cycle and relate these results to energy and macronutrient intakes. No significant differences were noted in snack and fruit/vegetable points, snack and fruit/vegetable button presses, percentage of snack points earned and fruit/vegetable intake, while only a trend was noted in preferred snack intake across the cycle. These results thus suggest that preferred foods varying in energy density may not necessarily be more reinforcing or sought after during certain phases of the menstrual cycle.

There are limitations to this study. The present findings are limited to a small sample, where the results of only 17 women were analysed. Direct measurements of energy and macronutrient intakes were only taken for 1 day (8h00-17h30) inside the laboratory for each phase. Evening snacking was also not measured on these days, meaning that we are unable to draw conclusions based on the direct assessment of 24-hour EI. Further measurements of appetite, including hunger and satiety, with VAS were not performed, limiting our interpretation of potential variations in appetite across the cycle.

In conclusion, no differences were noted in EI, macronutrient intakes, REE and PAEE across the menstrual cycle. The measurement of these factors within the same individuals provides a better idea of the non-significant variations in EI, REE and PAEE which occur across the menstrual cycle. Taken together, this suggests that the menstrual cycle may not be of practical concern when assessing food intake and physical activity patterns under the methodological conditions presented in this study.

Acknowledgments

The authors would like to thank the participants for their devoted participation. É. Doucet is a recipient of a CIHR/Merck-Frosst New Investigator Award, CFI/OIT New Opportunities Award and of an Early Research Award. The authors declare no conflict of interest.

References

[1] Dye L and Blundell JE (1997) Menstrual cycle and appetite control: implications for weight regulation. *Hum. Reprod.* 12, 1142-1151.

[2]   Johnson WG, Corrigan SA, Lemmon CR, Bergeron KB and Crusco AH (1994) Energy regulation over the menstrual cycle. *Physiol. Behav.* 56, 523-527.

[3]   Li ET, Tsang LB and Lui SS (1999) Menstrual cycle and voluntary food intake in young Chinese women. *Appetite* 33, 109-118.

[4]   Lyons PM, Truswell AS, Mira M, Vizzard J and Abraham SF (1989) Reduction of food intake in the ovulatory phase of the menstrual cycle. *Am. J. Clin. Nutr.* 49, 1164-1168.

[5]   Tarasuk V and Beaton GH (1991) Menstrual-cycle patterns in energy and macronutrient intake. *Am. J. Clin. Nutr.* 53, 442-447.

[6]   Dalvit-McPhillips SP (1983) The effect of the human menstrual cycle on nutrient intake. *Physiol. Behav.* 31, 209-212.

[7]   Martini MC, Lampe JW, Slavin JL and Kurzer MS (1994) Effect of the menstrual cycle on energy and nutrient intake. *Am. J. Clin. Nutr.* 60, 895-899.

[8]   Solomon SJ, Kurzer MS and Calloway DH (1982) Menstrual cycle and basal metabolic rate in women. *Am. J. Clin. Nutr.* 36, 611-616.

[9]   Riad-Gabriel MG, Jinagouda SD, Sharma A, Boyadjian R and Saad MF (1998) Changes in plasma leptin during the menstrual cycle. *Eur. J. Endocrinol.* 139, 528-531.

[10]   Angst J, Sellaro R, Merikangas KR and Endicott J (2001) The epidemiology of perimenstrual psychological symptoms. *Acta Psychiatr Scand* 104, 110-116.

[11]   Both-Orthman B, Rubinow DR, Hoban MC, Malley J and Grover GN (1988) Menstrual cycle phase-related changes in appetite in patients with premenstrual syndrome and in control subjects. *Am. J. Psychiatry* 145, 628-631.

[12]   Dye L, Warner P and Bancroft J (1995) Food craving during the menstrual cycle and its relationship to stress, happiness of relationship and depression; a preliminary enquiry. *J. Affect Disord.* 34, 157-164.

[13]   Lappalainen R and Epstein LH (1990) A behavioral economics analysis of food choice in humans. *Appetite* 14, 81-93.

[14]   Frank TC, Kim GL, Krzemien A and Van Vugt DA (2010) Effect of menstrual cycle phase on corticolimbic brain activation by visual food cues. *Brain Res.* 1363, 81-92.

[15]   Murphy KG and Bloom SR (2004) Gut hormones in the control of appetite. *Exp. Physiol.* 89, 507-516.

[16] Al-Harithy RN, Al-Doghaither H and Abualnaja K (2006) Correlation of leptin and sex hormones with endocrine changes in healthy Saudi women of different body weights. *Ann. Saudi Med.* 26, 110-115.

[17] Hardie L, Trayhurn P, Abramovich D and Fowler P (1997) Circulating leptin in women: a longitudinal study in the menstrual cycle and during pregnancy. *Clin. Endocrinol. (Oxf)* 47, 101-106.

[18] Mannucci E, Ognibene A, Becorpi A, Cremasco F, Pellegrini S, Ottanelli S, Rizzello SM, Massi G, Messeri G and Rotella CM (1998) Relationship between leptin and oestrogens in healthy women. *Eur. J. Endocrinol.* 139, 198-201.

[19] Thong FS, McLean C and Graham TE (2000) Plasma leptin in female athletes: relationship with body fat, reproductive, nutritional, and endocrine factors. *J. Appl. Physiol.* 88, 2037-2044.

[20] Bermant G and Davidson JM (1974) *The biological bases of sexual behavior.* New York: Harper Row.

[21] McNeil J, Riou ME, Razmjou S, Cadieux S and Doucet E (2012) Reproducibility of a food menu to measure energy and macronutrient intakes in a laboratory and under real-life conditions. *Br. J. Nutr.*, 1-9.

[22] Bingham SA, Cassidy A, Cole TJ, Welch A, Runswick SA, Black AE, Thurnham D, Bates C, Khaw KT, Key TJ and et al. (1995) Validation of weighed records and other methods of dietary assessment using the 24 h urine nitrogen technique and other biological markers. *Br. J. Nutr.* 73, 531-550.

[23] Flint A, Raben A, Blundell JE and Astrup A (2000) Reproducibility, power and validity of visual analogue scales in assessment of appetite sensations in single test meal studies. *Int. J. Obes. Relat. Metab. Disord.* 24, 38-48.

[24] Bouten CV, Sauren AA, Verduin M and Janssen JD (1997) Effects of placement and orientation of body-fixed accelerometers on the assessment of energy expenditure during walking. *Med. Biol. Eng. Comput.* 35, 50-56.

[25] Goris AH, Meijer EP, Kester A and Westerterp KR (2001) Use of a triaxial accelerometer to validate reported food intakes. *Am. J. Clin. Nutr.* 73, 549-553.

[26] Allen SS, McBride CM and Pirie PL (1991) The shortened premenstrual assessment form. *J. Reprod. Med.* 36, 769-772.

[27] Saelens BE and Epstein LH (1996) Reinforcing value of food in obese and non-obese women. *Appetite* 27, 41-50.

[28] Johnson WG, Carr-Nangle RE and Bergeron KC (1995) Macronutrient intake, eating habits, and exercise as moderators of menstrual distress in healthy women. *Psychosom Med.* 57, 324-330.

[29] Frye CA and Demolar GL (1994) Menstrual cycle and sex differences influence salt preference. *Physiol. Behav.* 55, 193-197.

[30] Brennan IM, Feltrin KL, Nair NS, Hausken T, Little TJ, Gentilcore D, Wishart JM, Jones KL, Horowitz M and Feinle-Bisset C (2009) Effects of the phases of the menstrual cycle on gastric emptying, glycemia, plasma GLP-1 and insulin, and energy intake in healthy lean women. *Am J. Physiol. Gastrointest Liver Physiol.* 297, G602-610.

[31] Gong EJ, Garrel D and Calloway DH (1989) Menstrual cycle and voluntary food intake. *Am. J. Clin. Nutr.* 49, 252-258.

[32] Lissner L, Stevens J, Levitsky DA, Rasmussen KM and Strupp BJ (1988) Variation in energy intake during the menstrual cycle: implications for food-intake research. *Am. J. Clin. Nutr.* 48, 956-962.

[33] Fong AK and Kretsch MJ (1993) Changes in dietary intake, urinary nitrogen, and urinary volume across the menstrual cycle. *Am. J. Clin. Nutr.* 57, 43-46.

[34] Capobianco G, de Muro P, Cherchi GM, Formato M, Lepedda AJ, Cigliano A, Zinellu E, Dessole F, Gordini L and Dessole S (2010) Plasma levels of C-reactive protein, leptin and glycosaminoglycans during spontaneous menstrual cycle: differences between ovulatory and anovulatory cycles. *Arch. Gynecol. Obstet.* 282, 207-213.

[35] Mills PJ, Ziegler MG and Morrison TA (1998) Leptin is related to epinephrine levels but not reproductive hormone levels in cycling African-American and Caucasian women. *Life Sci.* 63, 617-623.

[36] Teirmaa T, Luukkaa V, Rouru J, Koulu M and Huupponen R (1998) Correlation between circulating leptin and luteinizing hormone during the menstrual cycle in normal-weight women. *Eur. J. Endocrinol.* 139, 190-194.

[37] Cross GB, Marley J, Miles H and Willson K (2001) Changes in nutrient intake during the menstrual cycle of overweight women with premenstrual syndrome. *Br. J. Nutr.* 85, 475-482.

[38] Bryant M, Truesdale KP and Dye L (2006) Modest changes in dietary intake across the menstrual cycle: implications for food intake research. *Br. J. Nutr.* 96, 888-894.

Index

D

E

F

T